THE DISPENSARIES

Healthcare for the
Poor Before the NHS

Britain's Forgotten Health-care System

Michael Whitfield

authorHOUSE®

AuthorHouse™ UK
1663 Liberty Drive
Bloomington, IN 47403 USA
www.authorhouse.co.uk
Phone: 0800.197.4150

Published by AuthorHouse 04/20/2016

ISBN: 978-1-5049-9716-4 (sc)
ISBN: 978-1-5049-9715-7 (hc)
ISBN: 978-1-5049-9717-1 (e)

Print information available on the last page.

Any people depicted in stock imagery provided by Thinkstock are models,
and such images are being used for illustrative purposes only.
Certain stock imagery © Thinkstock.

This book is printed on acid-free paper.

Because of the dynamic nature of the Internet, any web addresses or links contained in
this book may have changed since publication and may no longer be valid. The views
expressed in this work are solely those of the author and do not necessarily reflect the
views of the publisher, and the publisher hereby disclaims any responsibility for them.

Front cover photograph is of the Clifton Dispensary, Bristol with a small copy of Dr Lettsom's
drawing to illustrate his home visit in 1780 (see page 96), courtesy Wellcome library.

CONTENTS

PREFACE

The British National Health Service (NHS) is in crisis. After more than sixty years of a government-run and -funded health service, which was brought in by the Labour Party in 1946, all is not well. Most of the hospital trusts are running huge deficits, the morale of the staff is low, and there is no clear political solution to the problem. The original aim of providing a comprehensive 'free at the point of need service for medical problems' has been retained, but is being eroded at the edges, and many patients still opt for private consultations and treatment rather than face increasingly long waits and often impersonal care. The relationship between the medical profession and the government is at an all-time low, with the government attempting to control working conditions of the profession and quality of care.

Each new government attempts to introduce change in how the NHS is managed, which frustrates the health service staff as they try to deal with these changes. Most health service workers and their patients have no knowledge of how illness was managed before the NHS came into being. This book was written to describe how people coped with medical problems during the two hundred years before the start of the NHS.

For centuries, people have tried to find ways to help others who have been affected by serious diseases. Hospitals and infirmaries were built in cities and towns to look after people with serious diseases and accidents, and in many cases, general practitioners run their surgeries in small premises scattered throughout our towns and villages.

Hospitals and general practitioners existed for many years before the NHS, but there was also another sort of institution that helped manage illness: the dispensary. The word 'dispensary' has changed in meaning over the last two or three centuries. Nowadays it means a place or room where drugs are stored, made up according to prescriptions, and dispensed, such as in some rural general practices and in hospitals.

In the past, however, a dispensary was a charitable institution where medicines were dispensed, and medical advice was given freely or for a small charge. These charitable institutions were a key part of health care during the late eighteenth, nineteenth, and twentieth centuries and have largely been forgotten, having been subsumed within the NHS, which was introduced in 1948. Little has been written about dispensaries, even though the buildings that housed them are still present in many towns throughout the United Kingdom. Zachary Cope[1] suggested the reason for the paucity of literature is because there was never a national union or association of dispensaries formed in Britain. Failing such an association, there was no common purpose or propaganda, no annual conference at which the work of the various institutions could be discussed and publicised, and no representative body which, at the critical stage of their existence, could give the united experience and views of those who had the greatest and most valuable knowledge of their working.

Under the National Health Service Act of 1946, most of the country's medical buildings were transferred to the NHS. This included most voluntary hospitals, clinics, and dispensaries. From the beginning of the NHS, patients were freely cared for by hospitals, general practitioners. and the public health services.

Dispensaries funded by subscriptions disappeared overnight. Those institutions run by subscribers were no longer needed. The subscriber system of funding institutions to look after the medical problems of the poor, where the subscriber has the right to introduce the patient to the dispensary or the voluntary hospital by handing over a note, is an historical oddity. It ensured that the wealthy donor developed a relationship with the poor patient, even though the relationship may not have lasted a long time. In many ways, a relationship like this can be considered appropriate and will have brought many wealthy people knowledge of the problems faced by the poor; but on the other hand, this sort of dependent relationship can be seen as inappropriate and demeaning. The notes or tickets would have been handed to the 'deserving' poor, rather than paupers and beggars who would most likely have been directed to the poorhouse. Patients were not supposed to make use of dispensaries if they could afford to pay doctors for the care of family members and their servants. Deciding whether they could afford to pay was largely left to the subscribers who provided the notes. Doctors working in the dispensaries sometimes resented seeing patients when it seemed the patients had adequate resources to pay for treatment.

The dispensaries developed because they were economical compared to the cost of running hospitals and they provided care for those patients too sick to travel to hospitals and finally, working in a dispensary provided a doctor with an unrivalled opportunity for the study of disease and self-promotion. Loudon[2] suggests that had the voluntary hospitals of the eighteenth and early nineteenth centuries expanded, particularly in the outpatient departments, the dispensaries might never have been founded.

The dispensary doctors looked after many illnesses and people who would not have been treated in the hospitals. According to the third annual report of the Gloucester Dispensary (1834): 'Smallpox, scarlatina, and other cases of a dangerous description and some requiring serious operations have occurred where the patients have been unable to leave their homes ... cases utterly hopeless as to ultimate cure, but in which medicine may mitigate the sufferings of the patient and smooth, in some degree, the passage to the grave. Many such cases were admitted annually under the care of the dispensary'.

Children younger than six or seven were not admitted to hospitals in the early parts of the nineteenth century. Infectious diseases were feared by the voluntary hospitals, so if the patient was feverish or had a rash or looked as if he might have diarrhoea and or vomiting, the patient was viewed with great suspicion and almost certainly not admitted. The last thing hospital authorities wanted was an outbreak of an infectious disease in the confined situation of a hospital.

If a poor person was too weak to leave his or her home, the dispensary doctors would visit to diagnose and treat the problem, provided the patient lived within a carefully circumscribed area around the dispensary and was able to procure a note from a subscriber. If these conditions were not met, the patient had no alternative but to seek help from the Poor Law provision, which after 1834 usually meant admission to a workhouse. Most of the dispensary doctors lived in the same area as their patients, and many remained in their post for many years. The resident doctors were full-time employees of the dispensaries and were often precluded from taking private patients, especially during their first few years of employment. Some used these posts as steps to future higher office, but all gained considerable experience of home visiting and the sort of life lived by the poor that would not have been gained by doctors following traditional private practice.

Particularly towards the second half of the nineteenth century, many doctors got involved with the provident system, where patients were encouraged to regularly pay a small sum to ensure that they could get care when it was needed. It was an insurance system that ensured patients obtained predetermined levels of care.

Reading about management issues in dispensaries, such as the challenges of appointing suitable doctors, ensuring that they worked appropriately and didn't delegate their work inappropriately to assistants, and ensuring that they informed the committee if they took on private patients or moved outside the catchment area reminds me of issues surrounding the management of salaried doctors today. There is little doubt that some doctors are difficult to manage! And it's easy to see why some value their self-employed status. Management of the profession before the NHS started was done very differently from how the government is attempting to control doctors nowadays.

This book starts with the Bristol dispensaries. As the second largest provincial town in England in 1700 and fourth-largest in 1801, it is a good place to start, especially as the city prided itself that it had long stood at the head of all other cities, for the number, magnitude, and diversity of its benevolent institutions. The city was one of the first to establish a public Infirmary and had numerous dispensaries. In 1801 the population of Bristol was about 61,000, and by 1901 it had risen to about 359,000. Despite the loss of many records relating to these dispensaries from bombing during World War 2, detailed investigation of the remaining dispensary records illustrates many of the features of these important institutions that provided health care to the poor.

LIST OF TABLES

ACKNOWLEDGEMENTS

In writing this book, I'm very grateful for the enormous amount of help I received from librarians and archivists, particularly those attached to the Bristol Record Office, the Bristol Reference Library, and the Special Collections of the University of Bristol. The Wellcome Library in London also provided me with much useful information.

On a personal level, Julian LeGrand, John Wilmot, and Barry Williamson have helped me in various ways, but any errors and conclusions are mine. Mavis, as always, has been supportive and put up with much as I pursued this subject. I am highly grateful to them all.

Chapter 1

AN INTRODUCTION TO THE BRISTOL DISPENSARIES

Two hundred years ago, Bristol, like most large cities, was an unhealthy place. There were two hospitals, the Infirmary and St Peter's, and about two hundred doctors. Most Bristol citizens tried to have nothing to do with either hospital care or the doctors, for hospitals had little to offer in the way of a cure, and doctors' remedies often made things worse. Life expectancy was short; few reached forty years of age, and the infant mortality rate was high. Most of the population died of infectious diseases like smallpox, typhoid, and cholera, as well as respiratory diseases such as tuberculosis and pneumonia, and many women died giving birth. Medical care, as now, was expensive (in those days the costs were mostly doctors' fees, whereas now the costs of medicine and surgery form the largest cost of medical treatment by far).

Much has been written about Bristol's hospitals but little about the other institutions, particularly the dispensaries, that were created in the nineteenth century to relieve sickness. The dispensaries were not simply places to provide medicines; they were more like our modern-day health centres but had many significant differences from these important parts of our National Health Service. Hodgkinson[3] commented that the development of dispensaries should have been fostered and guided from above but was left to ad hoc invention and management as inclination

1

dictated. The early part of this book describes the development of dispensaries in Bristol, a development that provided a large British city with a system of medical care that was totally wiped away with the institution of the National Health Service in 1948.

In 1750, a poor family with a sick child faced an unenviable choice: with no money to pay any form of healer, they were left to select practitioners they could afford, even ones with no qualifications except perhaps years of experience. Their local reputation, good or bad, didn't matter. There were no hospitals or clinics that would accept the care of a child. Home remedies were usually resorted to, and that was about all poor families could choose from.[4]

In the main, dispensaries were created to provide medical care for the poor of the city. Most dispensaries were developed and supported by wealthy citizens who exerted a system of control on how they were to be used. The development of dispensaries can be seen as an alternative to the Poor Law provisions, the large voluntary hospitals, and the local doctors. The list of Bristol dispensaries can be seen in Table 1.

Table 1   The Bristol Dispensaries

Name of Dispensary	Year Established
John Wesley's Dispensary, New Room, Broadmead	1746
The Bristol Dispensary	1775
Thomas Beddoes' Dispensary Dowry Square	1799
Thomas Beddoes' Dispensary, Little Tower Court, Broad Quay	1803
Prichard's Dispensary Castle Green	1810
Bristol Eye Dispensary	1811
Clifton Dispensary	1814
Redcliffe Street Dispensary	1814
Institution for the Cure of Diseases of Children	1826
Skin Dispensary	1846
Institute for the Cure of Deafness and Diseases of the Ear	1851
Homoeopathic Dispensary, Queen Square (later Upper Berkeley Place)	1852

Homoeopathic Dispensary, The Triangle, Clifton	1853
Free Institution for the Care of Women and Children	1857
Redland Dispensary	1860
General Dispensary for Children, Redland	1870
Forester's Medical Institute	1873
Read Dispensary for Women and Children	1874
Bristol Provident Dispensaries, Hotwells, Barton Hill, St Phillips, Cheltenham Road, Bedminster	1876
Institute for Skin and General Diseases	1883
Homoeopathic Dispensary, Brunswick Square	1883

Records about the first dispensary in Bristol in 1746 are scarce, but such as they are, they indicate that it was the creation of the Wesleyan Methodists, and John Wesley's small book *Primitive Physic* was produced 'to help the dispensary work'. The New Room in Bristol was built by John Wesley in Broadmead in 1739, primarily as a preaching house, but it also housed a school for poor children and a dispensary with free medicine for the poor.[5] By January 1747, the number of patients attending this dispensary was given as two hundred. It closed shortly afterwards as Wesley had difficulty in obtaining suitable medicines, possibly because the apothecaries were not willing to supply them.

By the beginning of the nineteenth century, dispensaries had been created in many parts of London and in many provincial towns. Loudon described sixteen dispensaries in London and twenty-two throughout England,[6] with the Bristol Dispensary being formed second to the one in Stroud, Gloucestershire.

One of the best known medical men in Bristol at this time, Thomas Beddoes, who ran his own dispensary in Dowry Square, Clifton, from 1799, wrote:

> Dispensaries might easily be established in every town, and by means of dispensaries, medicines might be distributed with equal advantage as to economy, and with much greater convenience to patients. If physicians are needed, it would be much cheaper, by

paying them for their attendance at stated times and place, to bring physicians to patients than to build a hospital on purpose to bring patients to physicians. And what adds force to this observation, is that the most important acute diseases and those which require frequent visitation, are necessarily excluded from hospitals by their contagious nature.[7]

Beddoes was one of Bristol's most eminent physicians but, perhaps surprisingly, was never appointed to the staff of a hospital. He ran two dispensaries in Bristol, the other being in Little Tower Court, Broad Quay, which started in 1803. His 'Rules of the Medical Institution for the Sick and Drooping Poor' drew the comment from a reviewer in *The Medical and Physical Journal*:

'[T]here is something truly original in everything that comes from the hand of Dr Beddoes'.[8] Beddoes encouraged the poor to have sensible ways of living such as to 'contrive to stop the crevices and panes for a time, or find some snug corner for new born babies', and encouraged families to 'have as many beds as they could provide'. His truly original idea in the Rules was his insistence of a deposit of two shillings and sixpence for every patient, that was handed back to the patient at the end of their treatment. As he wrote: 'The experience of former medical charities shows that the sick are constantly flying off before they have a chance of due benefit. I take this to be a want of proper understanding'.

There were two main dispensaries in Bristol in the nineteenth and twentieth centuries. The largest was the Bristol Dispensary, which was situated near the centre of Bristol and started in 1776. In the Bristol Dispensary's annual report of 1776, the committee attempted to justify its role in the health care of Bristol. This justification was clearly centred on the Christian maxim that it is more blessed to give than to receive, and the need to relieve those in sickness and poverty.

'Can there be a more exalted pleasure to the truly benevolent and humane than to visit such houses of distress, to step into them as angels of God for good, to rescue their miserable inhabitants from the complicated evils under which they groan, to administer to them the healing balm and to revive their dropping hearts and cause them to sing for joy?'[9]

The dispensary was designed to serve those poor who were unable to access care in the Infirmary, either as an outpatient or by being admitted. Although set up to care for those who were not able to be treated by the Infirmary, the dispensary too had rules about who could be treated. Patients had to live within a prescribed area of the city, and pregnant women had to prove they were married. As in the Infirmary, patients with venereal diseases were not accepted.

Table 2   Number of Patients Attending the Bristol Dispensary

Year	No. of patients seen	No. of deliveries	No. of doctors
1796	632		1
1807	2008	467	2
1816	1840	861	2
1826	2553	430	2
1836	1781		2
1856	3486	293	3
1861	4772	381	4
1872	6971	421	5
1874	8419	522	6

Hidden in surgeon Richard Smith's scrapbook records of the Bristol Infirmary is a handwritten letter from John Brent Cross to Smith[10] about an alternative dispensary. Cross states that the institution could only have existed in a room in Castle Green from 1810–11, as the founder was elected to St Peter's in 1811. The note ends by saying, 'I trust, my dear sir, that you did not think I had forgotten you; the fact is, I did not see Prichard until very lately, not choosing to excite his curiosity by calling to make enquiries. Details of the dispensary is confirmed in a letter describing the early biography of JC Prichard'.[11]

Dr James Cowles Prichard was a physician colleague of Smith's and is nowadays remembered as the owner of the Red Lodge in Park Row, Bristol, but he was one of the most influential physicians the Infirmary had ever had. His views and experiences as a physician newly arrived in Bristol are described below in a printed document signed by three eminent Bristol gentlemen but were obviously not shared by his colleagues.

> The dispensary is a very useful institution, yet it leaves many wants unprovided for. According to the established plan of the Bristol Dispensary, an apothecary prescribes for the great majority of the patients, and only calls in the aid of the physician when he deems it advisable. This practice is contrary to the routine of the dispensaries in London, Liverpool, and other large towns, where the physician prescribes for every patient. Some benefits are probably obtained by this peculiarity, but disadvantages are also attendant. At least a department is left void, which may be filled up with good effect.
>
> Influenced by considerations of this kind, the physician who ventures to make the present proposal, begun at the commencement of this year to give his advice to all poor persons who applied for it, at a place appointed in Castle Green. The prescriptions were compounded by a druggist and the medicines given to the patient gratis. No indirect application was required, that greater facility might be afforded, nor was any qualification made necessary except poverty and sickness. The experiment was then tried and the result verified the opinion which prompted

it. The resort of patients has been so considerable as to prove the want which was imagined to exist. The cases are recorded of 490 persons who have applied for and received medicines, since 8 January. That some benefit has actually been obtained is evident from the increasing number of applicants.

> In January 12 were admitted
> in Feb   22
> in March   32
> in April   43
> in May   78
> in June   103

The number is now greater than was at first expected; and the expense having become considerable, it is proposed to obtain the subscriptions of sixty to seventy persons annually, by which the cost of drugs may be defrayed. With this supply, it is computed that one hundred patients per month may receive medicines which will be dispensed on the most economical plan, according to certain formulae. Since the mere price of drugs will constitute the whole expense of the institution, it is evident that the sum collected will be spent in relieving a great relative proportion of sickness.

> Stewards
> Mr Joseph Storrs Fry
> Mr George Fisher
> Mr John Brent Cross

There are no other records about this experiment, and it looks as if it ceased working shortly after this letter was written.

The other large dispensary was the Clifton Dispensary, situated to the west of the city. This was created later and always remained smaller but appears to have taken Prichard's comments to heart, for the physicians clearly had a much more active role to play than in the Bristol Dispensary, particularly in the latter half of the nineteenth century and in the twentieth.

Table 3   Number of Patients Attending the Clifton Dispensary

Year	No of subscribers	No of patients seen	No of deliveries
1813	184	487	
1827		1752	
1859		2110	162
1878		2495	172
1900		3451	73
1920		1688	

Other dispensaries were started in Bristol during the nineteenth century, most following the initiative of one doctor. It is always difficult to know the motive behind such initiatives, but many were clearly a method of attracting patients. For example, in 1814, the Redcliffe Street Dispensary was opened by Dr Jordan (pupil to Mr Shannon, surgeon and man-midwife to the Middlesex Dispensary, London) for the relief of the poor and other afflicted at his house, No 84 Redcliffe Street, Bristol, where he gave advice to the poor gratis in all cases of physic and surgery from nine until twelve every morning, and from five until seven in the afternoon to others.

In his book *A Short History of Bristol General Hospital,* Symes mentioned that it was hoped that a dispensary might be attached to the Bristol General Hospital (opened in 1832) at a later date 'so that any mechanic, labourer, servant or other poor person, being unable to pay a surgeon or apothecary for attendance, might be admitted as an independent outpatient on procuring a recommendation from a subscriber or from two housekeepers; and on payment of 3s and 6d he was entitled to receive advice and medicines for six successive weeks'. This idea never flourished and was finally abandoned in 1840.[12]

What Did the State Provide for the Sick Poor?

The medical services provided under the state run Poor Law before 1834 varied throughout the country. The parish medical officers usually entered into a contract for attending the sick poor. They received very little pay for this and initially were exploited, as it was an open-ended contract, and in many areas the 'labouring poor' were trying to access medical care that was officially provided for the paupers. The Royal Commission into the operating of the Poor Laws of 1832 recommended an extension of workhouses and a reduction in what was termed 'outdoor relief', so that the paupers had to access the workhouses to get care, and the poor were encouraged to seek medical care from the voluntary dispensaries or to sell their few possessions to pay doctors.

After 1840, the Poor Law medical officer became the 'public vaccinator', adding to his already considerable duties. This action, though, resulted in a considerable reduction in the number of cases of smallpox.

Bristol's Poor Law medical provisions for the sick poor were unique and centred on St Peter's Hospital, which also served as the workhouse[13] that cared for sick paupers. Very elaborate rules and by-laws had accumulated over generations for running this institution, which was staffed by three honorary physicians and three honorary surgeons all elected in open competition. It was run by the Guardians of the Poor.

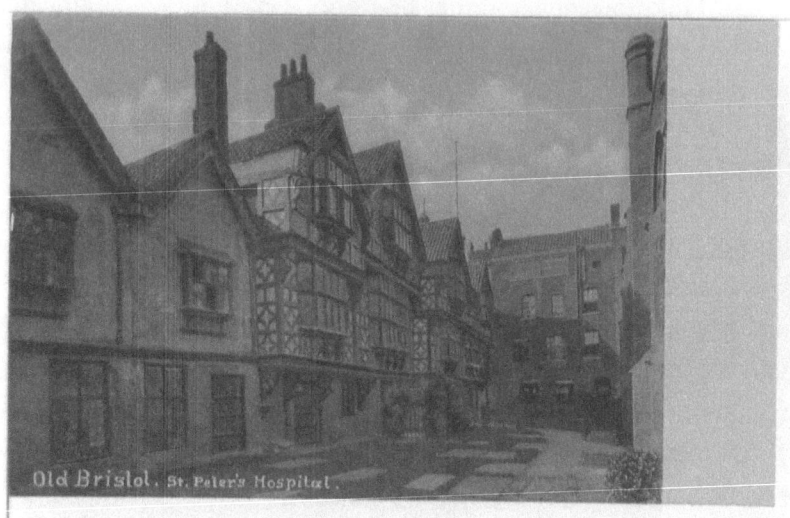

Old Bristol. St. Peter's Hospital.

St Peter's Hospital from Vaughan postcard
43207/9/27/13/3 courtesy Bristol Record Office

St Peter's Hospital

The doctors took turns being on duty a week at a time; each physician had to see his cases at least once a week and the surgeons three times a week. All emergencies had to be seen by the two duty doctors, and the doctors prescribed treatments that were dispensed by the resident apothecary. The apothecary was the only paid medical man of the Bristol Poor Law authorities, and he was employed full time and paid £120 per year. He had to be unmarried and live on the premises. He was never absent when the physicians and surgeons were visiting patients, nor was he allowed out after 11 p.m. without the permission of the governor of the workhouse. He was responsible for the accurate dispensing of medicines and was in charge of treatment. He had to keep the patients' case cards, which were fixed over every bed, up to date. A separate diary recorded all extraordinary cases. He also kept an outpatient book containing the names, addresses, diseases, and admission dates of every patient. He kept a similar book for inpatients. The apothecary was also responsible for drawing attention to any outbreak of infectious diseases in the wards.

The poor obtained medical relief by making an application to the apothecary, who was always in attendance on committee days. He wrote a note on each case and sent this to the committee. If applicants were recommended for admission into medical or surgical wards, a ticket was given to them addressed to the house steward.

Medicines were provided by the parochial authorities, and the average yearly cost of drugs was £235. In 1837, 1,200 cases were attended, which rose to 2,663 by 1844. Yet for this service the corporation paid only one doctor, although there were 64,000 inhabitants. In the middle of the nineteenth century, 72 per cent of pauperism resulted from sickness. In Bristol, 1,270 out of 2,200 cases received relief through sickness, in Clifton, 1,700 out of 2,600. These figures were given to the select committee of 1854 by Dr George Wallis, one of the Infirmary physicians.[14]

Wallis's Suggested Health Service for the Poor

In 1850 George Wallis published the book *Free Medical Aid to the Poor without Pauperism in Lieu of the Present Method of Poor Law Medical Relief*.[15] This little book suggested a system of medical care decades ahead of its time. The main suggestions include that

- A system of national free dispensaries shall be set up, which would be solely in the hands of medical officers appointed to the service as a distinct department of the Poor Law.
- The union surgeons and medical officers will form a corps called the Medical Civil Service under a director general. The corps will receive their pay by a salary without case payments. These salaries will depend on the duties performed. The boards of guardians shall provide all drugs, chemicals, medicines and remedies of all kinds. A proper place shall be provided in which the drugs etc. will be deposited as a dispensary, where the medical officer may prescribe for his patients.

- Every poor person shall be entitled to receive every medical or surgical aid he or she may require and which the medical or surgical officer may think necessary. It is deemed advisable to extend this assistance to the industrious and respectable poor, who are not paupers, to save them from being reduced to pauperism by sickness.

- All vagrants, trampers, and persons not of the district shall have medical or surgical assistance on the occurrence of any accident or illness, but the case shall be immediately referred to the relieving officer and placed under the control of the board of guardians to be dealt with as they see fit. But that person cannot be removed unless the medical officer certifies that the patient is safe to move.

- The board of guardians shall fix a limit in regards to wages or income to prevent people accessing the charity, but it shall not exclude any of the labouring population whose weekly wage do not exceed ten shillings a week. Remedies of any kind can only be continued for a week unless permission by the managing committee of the dispensary is given.

- The medical officer can choose a boy or man from among the paupers of the union house to be instructed and act as an assistant for five years at least. All patients shall be required to provide their own bottles, gallipots or receptacles, which should be clean and with corks, etc. Such receptacles can be provided, but a deposit will be required.

- Patients will be given a card indicating when he is required to return, and any patient using improper language to the medical officer shall be dismissed.

- All boards of guardians shall appoint annually a committee to manage the affairs of each district consisting of four guardians and two resident ratepayers. This committee to meet weekly and they shall inspect the names of every patient attending the dispensary. A properly educated and competent midwife will be employed.

- If a patient is incapable of visiting the dispensary, he shall make any application for a home visit before ten o'clock in the forenoon.
- The election of medical officers shall be elected by the board of guardians and then shall send the name to the physician in chief who can confirm or reject the appointment. Appointment is for seven years. The medical officer will supply patients with all necessary remedies, performance of vaccinations, operations in surgery, reducing and attending fractures and dislocations, and assisting the midwife in all difficult and dangerous cases. He will keep his statistical table, carefully recording all cases. Honorary physicians and surgeons may be appointed to any free national dispensary.
- Every union medical officer shall attend at his dispensary not less than three days in every week and on every day if the business of the district should require it.
- In all town districts one day in every week shall be specially appointed for the performance of vaccinations. The medical officer shall keep a journal of every difficult and dangerous case of midwifery to help determine whether the medical officer shall receive a gratuity.
- Infirmary wards should be maintained at every union to admit sick cases from the district dispensaries.

Wallis described the result of a practical experiment that was run in Bristol during the 1849 cholera epidemic. First, he described the epidemic of cholera in 1832. It prevailed for twelve weeks and two days, from 15 July to 9 October. There were 1521 cases of malignant cholera during the epidemic and 584 deaths. The expense of hiring medical officers was £460.

The cholera epidemic started on 10 June, 1849, and stopped on 16 October (eighteen weeks). This time there were 778 cases of cholera and 444 deaths. Wallis described how Bristol was divided into five districts, and a free dispensary was established in each district, a competent medical officer appointed to each. The total population of Bristol at the time was 64,266. More details about this epidemic can be found in *The Bristol Microscopists and the Cholera epidemic of 1849*.[16]

Wallis said the free dispensaries protected 25 per cent of the whole population, and fully two thirds of these were mechanics and labourers, not paupers. There were 7,000 paupers on the pay list.

He said, 'This is an important result of this system; the diarrhoea as cured by instant medical aid and the cases prevented from progressing into cholera, which is the usual course of the epidemic. An equally advantageous effect will be produced on all other acute diseases'.

The *British Medical Journal*[17] stated that Dr Wallis is widely known from his being adviser of a plan for ameliorating the present condition of the pauper population of the United Kingdom and by which plan he proposes to give to the poor every medical and surgical assistance, without them coming under the ban of pauperism. His plan was accepted by Mr C Buller, late president of the Poor Law board, who was about bringing in an Act fully carrying out the plan as a legislative measure, when, unfortunately, he died. Wallis was particularly distressed about this as he became aware that someone had taken his plan without acknowledgement and used it in Ireland.

In 1851 the Medical Charities (Dispensary) Act[18] placed Ireland's charitable dispensary system under the control of the Irish Poor Law Commission. Within each union, dispensary districts were formed, with a total of 723 being created across the country – an average of between four and five per union. The number of dispensaries operating was 960 in 1853, rising to 1,071 by 1872. Each district had its own dispensary where the poor could obtain free medicines and medical treatment from the dispensary medical officer, with the costs being borne by the boards of Guardians and funded through the poor rate.

Hodgkinson[19] concluded that trying to divorce the medical service from the Poor Law was the dominant theme of reformers in the 1850s. The inadequacy and the pauperising quality of the Poor Law medical service had taught many of the poor the advantages of self-help for the possibility of sickness. However, the continuing Poor Law provision provided in some parts of the country provided medical aid far superior to what the poor could provide for themselves.

Chapter 2

THE BRISTOL DISPENSARY

The Bristol Dispensary was founded in October 1775 and was established by Tabernacle Methodists, initiated by Revd T. Joss.[20] Miss Elisabeth Brain, the daughter of a surgeon and apothecary in Old Market, was the first treasurer but was soon replaced by Samuel Beck.

In 1942 the following article appeared in a Bristol newspaper[21]: 'Before the writer is a book, inscribed in neat handwriting. A journal of the rise and progress and proceedings of Ye Bristol Society for the Relief of Poor Persons when ill'.

It is a contemporary record of meetings, the names of those present, and a brief account of the business transacted. Here, for instance, are some of the entries relating to the meeting on November 20 1775 at the house of Mr Richard Sircom, on Castle Street:

'Resolved that Mr Mills is to furnish the society with a journal, cash book, and ledger.

'Resolved that Miss Brain, as treasurer, do give the maid at the Tabernacle House one shilling as a gratuity for cleaning the room'.

The last entry in this journal is as follows:

'We, whose names are underwritten, having fully and carefully investigated a complaint brought by John Neeve and his wife against Mr Williams for neglect in attendance of said John Neeve, do agree that Mr Williams is exculpated from the said charge. [Signed] Abe

Ludlow, John Wright, Joseph Fry, Robert Simpson, Robert Priest, Thos Shellard, JP Noble, and Morgan Yeatman'.

This is not dated, but the author adds, 'presumably John Wright was the founder of the Bristol printing firm [he wasn't, as he was one of the local physicians], and Joseph Fry was the doctor who founded the famous chocolate firm and that Robert Priest was the engineer whose firm, Priest and Mullins, still carries on in East Bristol'. Complaints against the staff of the dispensary over the next two hundred years were infrequent – but this was certainly the earliest!

The dispensary was modelled on the General Dispensary in Aldersgate Street in London that had been set up on the initiative of Dr John Lettsom (1744–1815).[22] Advice on the procuring of medical staff was offered by Lettsom, and there were two physicians, two surgeons, and two apothecaries. The surgeon and physician, Abraham Ludlow (1737–1807), played a particularly important role in the dispensary's activities.

In 1776 there were sixty subscribers, including Joseph Beck, the president and treasurer of the society, who was a prominent Quaker merchant, and Thomas Mills, a Quaker bookseller. Other subscribers included the mayor of Bristol, Andrew Pope; various doctors, including physicians John Wright and Abraham Ludlow; the apothecaries John Till-Adams, Robert Simpson, and William Williams; the man-midwife, John Castleman; Baptist minister Rev Caleb Evans; and Miss Elizabeth Brain, Mr Charles Whittuck (a Baptist associated with the Pithay meeting), Mr David Wait, Mr Isaacs, Mr Sircom, and Mr Martin, who were all involved in the initial Tabernacle Dispensary. Most subscribed one guinea a year, but Mr John Lewsley subscribed five guineas in the first year, JK Wilson, Esq., ten guineas. At least two of the doctors, Abraham Ludlow and John Till-Adams, were also Quakers. The subscription of one guinea meant the subscriber was entitled to have one medical patient at a time upon the list throughout the year and one lying-in, or pregnant, patient. During 1776, the dispensary looked after 175 patients, 115 being cured, 23 relieved, 14 discharged as incurable, and 16 who died.

The diary of the Quaker Sarah Fox[23] gives much information about these Quaker doctors and her own involvement with the dispensary. For instance, on 28 March 1793, she wrote that she had 'accompanied M. Beck to the dispensary committee. Found there able hands sufficient for the occasion'. John Till-Adams was described by her in January 1776 as 'a young apothecary lately come into considerable practice in Bristol, whence he had gone some years before to America with Bill Logan, and after his death returned with his widow to England. He had a good understanding and much medical knowledge and was now candidate for the affections of Nancy Fry'.[24] On 6 February 1779, Sarah dined with Till-Adams and was introduced to the subject of electricity, where she was prevailed upon to receive a shock and did not recover from the effects for several hours! On 20 February 1786, Till-Adams died.

Abraham Ludlow was born in 1737. He was the son of a Bristol surgeon and was appointed to the surgical staff of the Infirmary in 1767. Ludlow apparently ran into problems through treating medical cases in the Infirmary without holding an MD degree. In fact, he was prosecuted in the courts by his colleague Dr Rigge for doing so. Apparently, the case ended by him obtaining an MD and the following comment was made: 'The jury, being satisfied of his great abilities as a medical practitioner, did not enquire whether he had sent for it by post from Scotland, or whether like his opponent he had walked for it to Padua'.[25]

He was a man of immense activity and power of work; was one of the founders of the Bristol Library Society in 1772; kept a smallpox hospital in a house on Barton Hill; and inoculated patients with the help of John Ford and Dr Rodbard. He was described as 'having an imposing exterior. He moved with a measured step and affected a meditating abstraction of countenance, with a pomposity of diction and manners which could not but keep the vulgar at a respectable distance'.[26]

Sarah Fox describes visiting the inoculating house in 1768 with her nephew and niece: 'A very commodious house fitted for the reception of many patients and under good regulations. After the operation was performed, we brought them home till they sickened'.[27] This procedure was being done for several years before Edward Jenner published his work on the smallpox vaccination in 1796.

In 1781 a Mr Shelland and a Mr Carpenter were chosen as apothecaries, and it was established on 26 March of that year that 'all new apothecaries in future were to take the part of midwifery'. Shelland did not stay more than a year in this post. The average yearly income for the first ten years of the dispensary's existence was about £240–£250.

The annual report of 1792 included a list of the rules for the subscribers:

- Patients must not be able to attend the Infirmary or be able to pay for medical care. Every patient must have a recommendation from a subscriber. They must be residing within the boundary Temple Gate – Bedminster Causeway-west end of College Green – Fort Lane – St Michaels Hill – Stokes Croft – turnpike – Lawrence Hill Turnpike.
- Only married women who can produce a certificate or other proof of their marriage can be proper objects of this charity as midwifery patients.
- Sick patients within the boundary shall be admitted by the apothecary of the week and midwifery patients apply to the women's committee one month at least before they expect to lie-in. The committee meets fortnightly at Mr Wm Jordans in Wine street at half past ten in the morning precisely.

In that year there were 274 subscriptions of mostly one or two guineas. The staff of the dispensary included Doctors Ludlow and Wright as physicians to the dispensary to be consulted by apothecaries in extraordinary cases. The men-midwives to the dispensary were Mr John Castelman in extraordinary cases, and Mr Robert Simpson and Mr Thomas Rich. The apothecaries to the dispensary were Mr Robert Simpson, Castle Street, a Quaker, and Mr Thomas Rich, Broadmead.

In 1801 the dispensary was offering free vaccination for children with cowpox, and in 1813, the dispensary saw 784 midwifery cases and 1607 sick persons.

Table 4   Number of patients seen in the dispensary during one year in every decade[28]:

Year	Patients seen	Women delivered
1776	175	(In six years, 994 delivered)
1786	572	
1796	632	
1807	2008	467
1816	1840	861
1826	2553	430
1836	1781	

What Sort of Patients Were Being Seen at the Dispensary?

Rolfe, one of the apothecaries who started work in 1794, classified the problems he saw in 1800 and Loudon,[29] composed a table comparing Rolfe's findings with the diseases being seen at the Infirmary in the same year.

Table 5   Comparison of Cases seen in Bristol Dispensary and Bristol Infirmary in 1800

Bristol Dispensary Year 1800			Bristol Infirmary Outpatients Year 1800		
	No	Per cent		No	Per cent
Medical cases	939	98.5	Medical cases	786	79.6
Typhus, continued and putrid fevers	367	38.5	Typhus	1	
Other infective disorders	71	7.5	Other infective disorders	138	13.9

Mental disorders	15	1.6	Nervous disorders	25	2.5
Dropsy	33	3.5	Hydrops and anasarca	17	1.7
Respiratory disorders	158	16.6	Respiratory disorders	133	13.5
Phthisis	73		Phthisis	23	
Gastrointestinal disorders	188	19.7	Gastrointestinal disorders	118	11.9
Incl. dysentery and diarrhoea	114		Incl. dysentery and diarrhoea	64	
Genitourinary disorders	32	3.2	Genitourinary disorders	114	11.5
Skin diseases	0		Skin diseases	33	3.3
Diseases of locomotor system	24	2.5	Diseases of locomotor system	86	8.7
Other medical disorders	51	5.4	Other medical disorders	121	12.2
Surgical cases	14	1.5	Surgical cases	202	20.4
Inflammation and contusion	8		Inflammation and abscesses	29	
			Accidents	65	
			Leg ulcers	87	
Total	953			988	

Comparing mixes of diseases in the above way can only give a very rough approximation of what disease was seen in the two sites. However, it does seem surprising that not one patient with a skin disorder was seen at the dispensary. One of Bristol's physicians[30] wrote in 1820 that 'among the rules of the Bristol Infirmary, there is one which expressly forbids the admission of any patient labouring under contagious fever. For many years, however, this rule has been considered as indicating the ignorance or unreasonable timidity of those who enacted it … the house committee did not interfere and the records showed that during the epidemic, out of 2231 patients who received institutional care, 27 per cent were treated at the poor house [St Peter's Hospital], 29 per cent at the Infirmary [mostly outpatients], and 44 per cent at the dispensary'. In September 1807 the evangelical bookseller, Mills, resigned his position as secretary, having completed nearly thirty years in this post.

The Two Early Parts of the Dispensary

By 1807 the dispensary was divided into two districts with two buildings, one at 11 North Street, almost opposite The Full Moon Inn in Stokes Croft, and the other at 26 Bath Street, south of the river. Each district was under the care of an apothecary – John Jenkins being the apothecary of the northern district and Thomas Ashmeade of the southern district. By 1812, William Scott had taken over the southern district.

Both apothecaries became resident in his part of the dispensary. By 1816, the dispensary had been operating 41 years and had expanded. It now had a constituency that took in the area around the New Cut of the River Avon and the Hills and Harford bridges. The committee of the charity claimed that a total of 13,836 midwifery cases, and 41,436 sick cases had been attended to in the course of the charity's history. There were about 400 subscribers at this point.

With the great increase in numbers of patients, it was not surprising that by 1816, expenditure exceeded income by £150 during the year; by 1820, the continuing financial difficulty resulted in thoughts of closing one of the dispensaries. This did not happen, and by 1824 it was decided to replace the dispensary on Bath Street with one on Queen Square. The move to Queen Square was accomplished by purchasing the lease of 32 Queen Square for £200 – a large house on the southern side of the square, and by 1831, when the Bristol riots destroyed more than twenty-seven houses on Queen Square, the dispensaries were still caring for nearly two thousand patients and 460 pregnant women each year.

In 1826 John Earle was appointed apothecary of the Queen Square Dispensary, having been working in the North Street Dispensary, and remained there until 1843. However, in the 1841 census, he was not resident, being replaced by Dr Robert Watts, who subsequently became the resident medical officer of the Clifton Dispensary. William Scott, who was originally appointed apothecary of the Queen Square Dispensary in 1812, moved to North Street in 1812 and remained there until 1830.

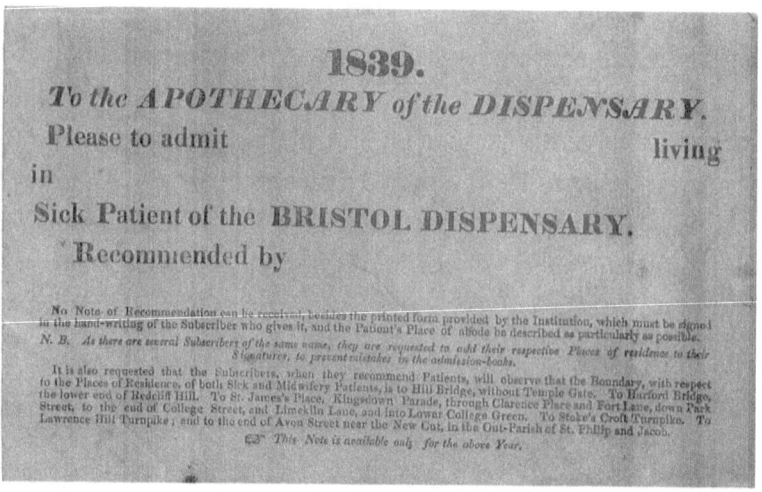

One of the 1839 notes that subscribers had to complete.[31]

Thomas Martin replaced John Earle in 1843 at the Queen Square Dispensary, which moved to 9 Queen Square in 1851.

In 1845 three dispensary doctors holding the qualification of Membership of the Royal College of Surgeons (MRCS) joined the many others in Bristol in criticising the college that had just introduced the new qualification of fellowship of the college. The three doctors were William Bird Herepath and William Smith, describing themselves as surgeon-accoucheurs to the Bristol Dispensary, and Robert Norton, describing himself as the apothecary to the Bristol Dispensary. The letter asserted that it was wrong of the council to introduce this new examination that would identify those with specialist surgical skills and separate surgeons into two classes.[32]

An example of how the dispensary was used in 1849.

In 1848, Dr William Smith and the Revd AT Pile, a local clergyman, were inspecting houses in the Hotwell district of Bristol. One house in Limekiln Lane (now St George's Road nearly opposite York Place) drew their attention. They found a closet situated just inside the front door, in a recess under the stairs. It was blocked and overflowing, the effects being as offensive as can be imagined. From time to time, attempts were made to clear the blockage using an iron rod, but this forced some of it beneath the house, into Webber's buildings, which from this cause had become uninhabitable. The doctor described how the closet was placed close to the only sitting room, and the partition being partially broken down, the effluvia pervaded the apartment – in fact, the whole house. A formal notice of the state of affairs was given to the authorities just before Christmas 1848, and a month later a reminder was given.

In February 1849 one of the children fell ill with a low-grade fever. Another clergyman gave the family a dispensary note, and under the care of the dispensary doctor, Dr Martin, the child fortunately and surprisingly recovered.

Dr Smith again complained about the blocked closet, but to no avail. On 1 May, he visited the premises with one of the Infirmary surgeons who was also a city councillor, and he found the contents of the tank still overflowing into the buildings below, next door to which nine cases of fever occurred about two years previously. The doctor had no hesitation in saying that more cases of fever will occur in that house or the neighbourhood, and obviously will entail an additional expense on the rate-payers during the ensuing summer, unless the nuisance was removed.[33]

In 1853, with more than 3000 patients being seen and 243 women delivered babies, it was decided that there was a need to appoint an additional medical officer, and a decision was also made to establish a central dispensary and to dispose of the two buildings on North Street and Queen Square. A building was found in Castle Green.

The Castle Green Dispensary

In 1858 the annual meeting reported that during that year, 291 poor lying-in women had been delivered, and 3,840 sick patients had been cured or relieved by means of the charity. The chairman reminded the subscribers that the regular income of the charity is not as yet equal to the expenditure.

Appointment of Doctors

The election of surgeons was done by the committee, and the following illustrates how Mr WT Winter was chosen in 1861.

They had received three applications for the post. 'Mr Whitwill, as knowing something of Mr Winter through the surgeon under whom he studied, proposed that he be appointed. The Rev D Cooper thought that as Mr Winter lived in the city and was the son of a respected minister, and was equally qualified with the other candidates, he should be given preference, unless a more qualified person arose'.[34]

In the 1861 census Mr Winter was aged 23 and lodging at 32 Queen Square. He resigned in 1866, and by 1871 was living in Westbury, Wiltshire.

In 1872 there were four medical officers, and they were seeing an increasing number of patients per week. In November 1873, 704 patients had been seen, but by December 1873, 378 patients were seen in one week.

In August 1873 it was decided to appoint an additional medical officer and to extend the area served by the dispensary to include Bedminster. Again, there were three applicants for the post, who was to get a salary of £150 per year for the first two years. One of the applicants withdrew as he could not accept the salary, and one of the other two was elected 7 to 3 by a show of hands. However, one of the subscribers demanded a poll on behalf of the unsuccessful candidate, and this man (Mr Hetling) was appointed a week later! He was the son of a former surgeon at the Infirmary.

In 1886[35] it was noted that two of the surgeons, Dr Robert Norton and Dr George Alexander Gloag, had resigned having served the Institution for sixteen years each. Robert Norton worked originally in the North Street Dispensary and in 1851 had lived in Castle Precincts and King Square subsequently. At the annual meeting it was mentioned that formerly it was the rule of the dispensary that no surgeon was allowed to enter private practice until he had served five years. Replacing the surgeons was now difficult in view of the small salary offered, and it was proposed to alter the rule to enable doctors to undertake private practice at the end of the first year.

Increasing Demand and the Introduction of the Provident Element

The centenary of the dispensary in 1876 was the beginning of a new phase in the administration of the charity. The annual report of that year[36] stated:

> 'The altered circumstances of the working classes render it desirable that the provident element should be introduced, as large numbers of those who seek the aid of the charity, although unable to encounter the entire charge of medical attendance, are well able to pay something towards the sick notes. However,

making the charity an entirely provident organisation could not be done, so the new rule was introduced. The reorganisation would slightly restrict the issue of "free notes" and promote the system of self-help among the working classes by calling upon those who can legitimately do so to contribute towards the expense of medical aid for which they apply:

'A subscriber of one guinea shall receive sick-notes, which may be given entire as free notes, or divided, and each half used as a note or recommendation, the patient paying half a crown (2s 6d) on presenting it at the dispensary; one midwifery note, available as a sick note; three notes of recommendation, entitling the bearer of each note to medical attendance on payment of six shillings on presentation at the dispensary'.

It was stated that the scheme is of a very modest character and some subscribers contended that it would hardly touch the evil system of pauperisation now going on. It was stated that no fewer than eighty thousand cases are gratuitously attended to every year by the medical activities of the city, and one speaker asserted that, within his own experience, many people earning 30 shillings and £2 a week refused to save a trifle for a time of sickness or distress, openly confessing that they looked to gratuitous medical help whenever it might be required. The new resolutions, however, were approved as an experiment, the committee holding out a prospect that the provident element should be further extended at a future time.

Two years later it was stated that 6,544 sick patients had been cured, and 377 lying-in women had been delivered. The annual report[37] stated that 'the work of the dispensary has decreased in the north-west portion of the city, but in the eastern and manufacturing neighbourhoods the demands yearly increases, and subscribers in Clifton would find their notes of infinite service in these localities'.

In 1880 it was reported that an enquiry had been received from a poor working man who wondered whether the committee would agree for two or three working men to subscribe and receive notes as one subscriber as there were many, like him, who would willingly pay a small sum. This suggestion was rejected as it would make 'the institution an opposition to the medical men in the city'.[38] The next year, at the express desire of the staff, an ophthalmic department was established and fitted with the necessary appliances, and Mr F Richardson Cross agreed to be the honorary surgeon.

The New Dispensary

The numbers using the dispensary were steadily increasing.[39]

Table 6   Numbers of patients and doctors from 1856-1874

Year	Number of doctors	Sick patients seen yearly	Midwifery patients
1856	3	3486	293
1861	4	4772	381
1872	5	6971	421
1874	6	8419	522

The dispensary premises in Castle Green in the early 1880s was a modified house and was proving utterly inadequate, so in 1886, some adjoining property was purchased from the corporation. The old premises were pulled down and the new premises, designed by Mr W Gough, were opened in 1888. The North Street premises were rented out and not sold until 1910 for £750.

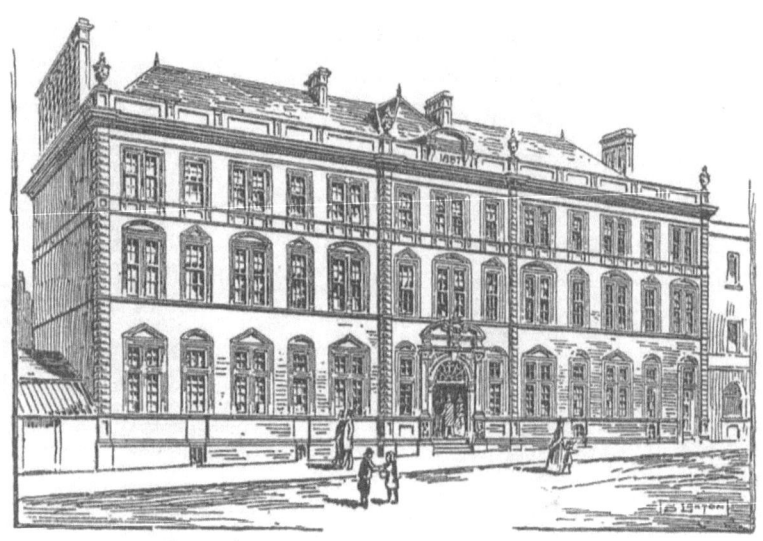

THE DISPENSARY, CASTLE GREEN; 1894.

Bristol Dispensary courtesy Bristol Central Library

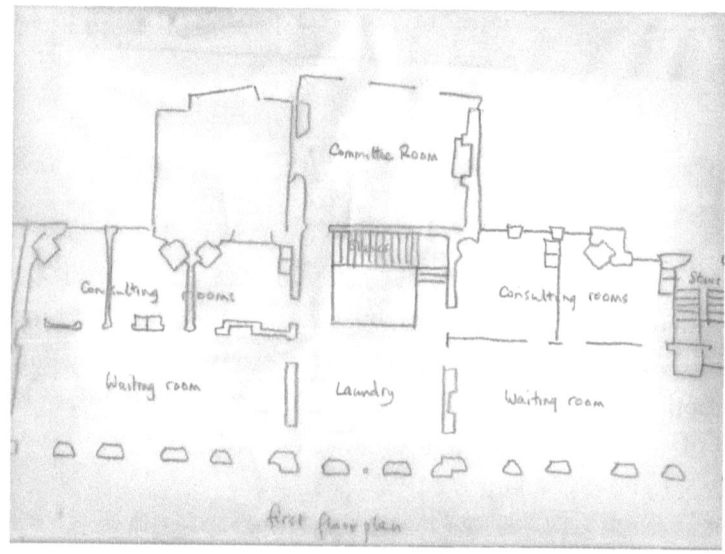

First Floor

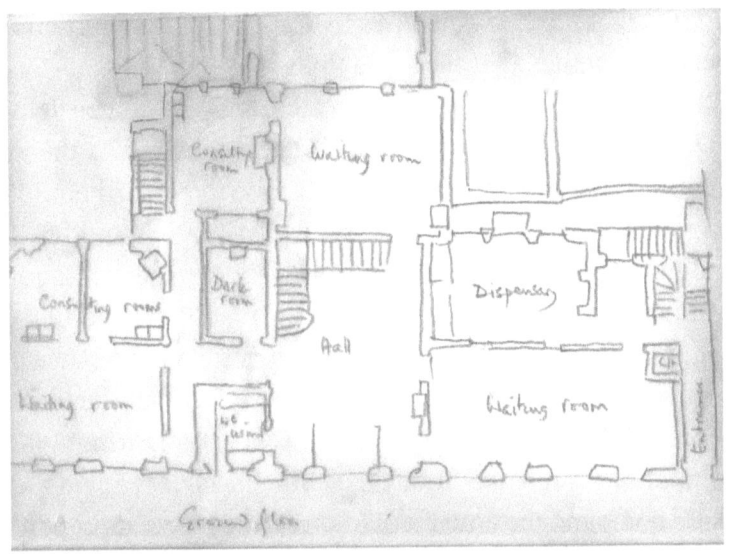

Ground Floor

Diagrammatic plans of the two lower floors
of the Castle Green Dispensary.[40]

The extensive basement contained cellars for coal and other materials and many toilets. The top floor was designed as a residence for one of the medical officers and a dispenser.[41] However, the top floor of the dispensary was allocated as living accommodation for the chief dispenser and his family and never housed a doctor. William Pollard and his family lived on the top floor of the dispensary from 1871 until after 1911, when he was seventy years old and still working.

The entrance hall and committee room of the new building had panelled wood ceilings that had been stained and varnished. The windows of the committee room were filled with ornamental stained glass. These windows had a shield in the upper portions containing the arms of Mr and Mrs Prideaux (the donors), those of the colleges of the physicians and surgeons, and those of the principal cities in the United Kingdom in which medical degrees were conferred. The buildings were entirely heated by gas stoves on a new system which warmed and ventilated at the same time.

In 1886, 8,142 patients had been treated, and 452 women delivered; in 1887 the figures were 8,142 and 452 respectively. At the annual meeting of the dispensary in 1888, Mr Fry, the chairman, told the meeting about the financial state of the charity: 'It should be borne in mind that for every guinea subscribed, six notes were issued, and the average cost of each note exceeded five shillings, so that every subscriber of a guinea was able to give to the sick poor what actually cost a guinea and a half. That arose from the fact that the institution has a considerable amount of funded property. During 1887, the subscriptions amounted to £1,717, including the amount paid for notes and share notes and the amount of interest from funded property was £1,200'.

Much information about the work of the dispensary can be obtained from the minutes of the Dispensary Committee from 1884 that were not destroyed during WW2.[42]

Table 7   Bristol Dispensary Medical Staff from 1884

Names	Qualifications	Year elected	Date resigned[R] or time expired [TE*]	
Dawson, Walter	MA, MB, Cantab	1884	1893	R
Page, George Shepley	LRCP, Edin	1885	1897	TE
Parker, George	MA, MD, Cantab	1887	1893	R
Cameron, John	MB, Glasgow	1888	1893	R
Maddison, WT	MD, Lond	1889	1904	TE
Powell, John Joseph	MD, Lond	1891	1903	R
Hill, Hedley	MRCS, LRCP	1891	1906	TE
Carling, Albert	MA, MB	1893	1908	TE
Hall, Elias George	MB, MRCS, Lond	1893	1908	TE
Webb, John Bartlett	MRCS, LRCP, Lond	1893	1908	TE

Leonard, Robert Cecil	MD, MRCS, LRCP	1897	1905	R
Phillips, C Morley	MD, MRCS, LRCP	1897	1907	R
Corfield, C	MRCS, LRCP	1903	1905	R
Moore, Leonard Augustine	MRCS, LRCP	1904	1918	TE
Newman, HRC	MB, MRCS, LRCP	1905	1925	TE
Richardson, AWC	MB, Lond	1906	1908	R
Coleridge, Alfred	MB, BS, Lond	1906	1911	R
Elliott, WHA	MB, BS, Lond	1907		
Bergin, Frank	MRCS, LRCP, Lond	1907		
Glenny, ET	MB, BS, Lond	1908	1908	R
Morris, LN	MRCS, LRCP	1908		
Pinniger, WJH	MD, Lond	1908	1910	R
Blackett, JF	MB, BS	1908	1910	R
Finzel, H	MD, Lond	1908		
Herepath, CEK	MD, Lond	1910		R
Dixon, Thomas Benjamin	MRCS, LRCP	1910		
Robertson, D	MB, ChB, Edin	1911		R
Page, Leonard	MRCS, LRCP	1919		
James, Charles Wanklyn	MRCS, LRCP	1919	1919	R
Zealand, Leo	MD, BA, Canada	1920		
Johnson, RG	MB, Lond	1920		
Elkington		1924		R
Evans	MB, ChB	1924		
Duerden, John R	MB, ChB	1925		
Davis, GM	MB, ChB	1927		
Perry, C Bruce	MB, ChB, Bristol MD, Lond	1929	1934	R
Moore, Hastings	MB, ChB	1932		

Myles, Q St Ledger	MA, MB, BCh, Oxon	1932
Evans, G Morton	MB, ChB	1934
Finzel HFM	MB, BS, Lond	1934
Matthews, R Amherst	MB, ChB, Bris	1934

*Time expired indicates that the doctor had been working at the dispensary for fifteen years – the maximum time allowed until 1923 when it was extended to twenty years.

The days for seeing outpatients were as follows (see map below for information about the areas of numbered districts):

No 1 City St Augustine and Kingsdown
Tuesday and Friday Dr Carling
No 2 St James, Stokes Croft, part of Kingsdown
Wednesday and Saturday Dr Powell
No 3 St Paul's, Newfoundland Rd and Ashley
Wednesday and Saturday Dr Maddison
No 4 Stapleton, Pennywell Roads
Tuesday Friday Dr Hall
No 5 St Judes, Newtown and Barton Hill
Monday and Thursday Mr Webb
No 6 St Phillips and The Marsh
Tuesday and Friday Mr Page
No 7 Temple, Redcliffe and Bedminster
Monday and Thursday Mr Hill

The expenditure of the dispensary in 1884 included cheques paid to medical officers for quarterly amounts of between £50 and £54 – secretary £25 and midwives £29.10. To indicate the approximate value of these figures, £1 in 1900 is equivalent to £57 in 2005 (e.g., a medical officer was being paid the equivalent of £11,400 per annum).

A site for the Malago Branch Dispensary in Bedminster was agreed on 8 Nov 1895, and this opened on 1 December 1897.

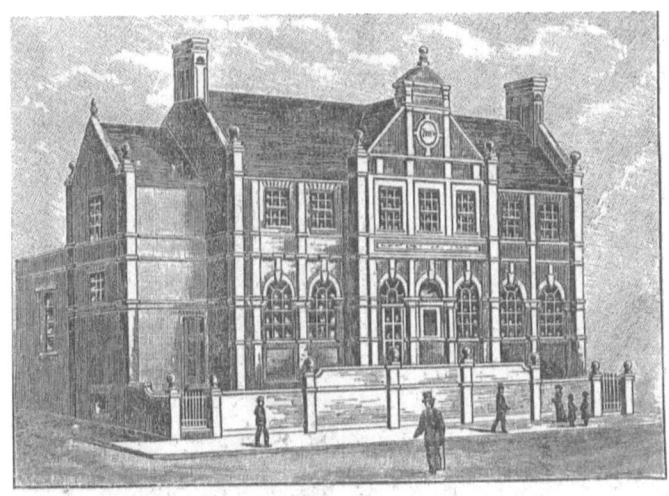

BEDMINSTER BRANCH OF THE BRISTOL DISPENSARY,
MALAGO ROAD, MILL LANE.

In November 1899 it was agreed that the medical officers should not be allowed to do private work until they had worked for the dispensary for two years – an increase from the previous one year.

The annual report of 1899 stated that attendances had continued to increase and arose from the increased use by the employees of large firms. These firms had been purchasing multiple subscriptions each year to enable this to happen, with private subscriptions declining. Mr FJ Fry of the Chocolate Firm, the treasurer, resigned, having been associated with the dispensary for forty-two years.

A request from University College had been received, indicating that a course of lectures for pupil midwives was being instituted at the college, and they wanted to know whether the committee of the dispensary would permit the pupils to attend cases under the supervision of the dispensary midwives. The question was referred to the medical officers, and the next month it was reported that the medical officers and the midwives agreed that they would not give permission for this to occur.

The Twentieth Century

By 1901, the number of doctors employed had increased to eight, and each had his own district (see map). The number of patients seen was 11,942 and 463 women were delivered.

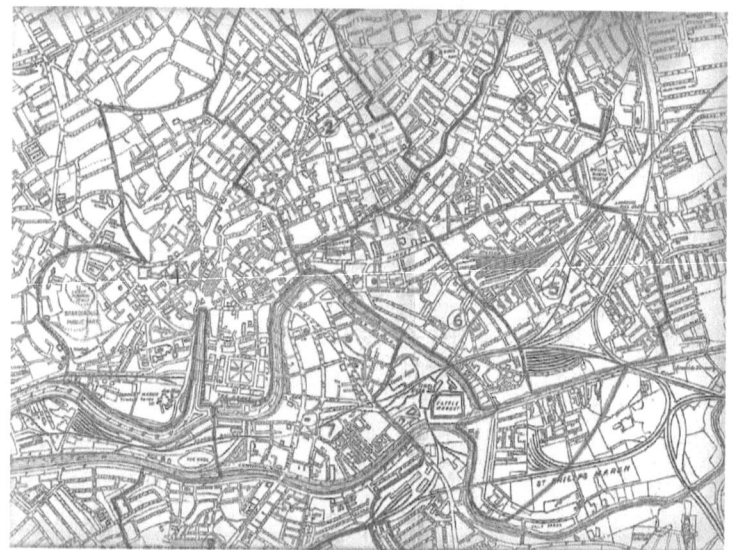

Map of Bristol indicating the visiting boundaries of
the Bristol Dispensary in 1901 with the dispensary
marked as a rectangle in section 6.
courtesy Bristol Record Office 33041 BMC/13/1-4

The doctors in 1901 were WT Maddison, MD, London, 1859–1923, an Irish doctor who practised from 172 Stapleton Road; John J Powell, MD, London, 1860–1943 who practised from 2 Portland Place; Hedley Hill, MD, Brux, 1868–1931, practising from Redcliffe; A Carling, MA, MB, Cantab, who lived in Great George Street from 1901; Elias George Hall, MB, London, who lived in Hampton Road, Redland, moving to Apsley Road, Clifton; John Bartlett Webb, MRCS, LRCP, London, who practised from Brunswick Square; RC Leonard, MD, Durham, the nephew of Crosby Leonard, one of the surgeons at the Infirmary; C Morley Phillips, MD, Brux, who remained single and lived in Ravenslea, Brislington.

The rules had evolved over the previous century and now a Subscriber received a book of notes containing five sick notes (which may be given entire as free notes, or divided, and each half used as a note of recommendation, the patient paying half a crown on presenting it at the dispensary), one midwifery note (which may be used as a sick note), and two notes of recommendation, entitling the bearer of each note to medical attendance on payment of five shillings.

A donation of £21 shall constitute a lifetime subscription and entitle the donor to the same privileges as an annual subscriber of one guinea. Annual subscriptions shall become due on 1 January each year.

As before, no patients with venereal complaints could be looked after, and patients properly recommended and residing within the boundaries were admitted daily – Sundays, Good Friday, Christmas Day, and bank holidays excepted – and would be attended by the surgeon in whose district they resided. No domestic servant could be visited as a patient in the home of his or her master or mistress, but such a servant could be admitted as a patient if able to attend at the dispensary.

No subscriber was permitted to recommend any member of his or her family.

Just over £2,000 was received from subscribers who now included many businesses, such as the Bristol Gas Company (ten subs), Bristol Sanitary Authority (seventy subs), JS Fry and Sons (120 subs), ES and A Robinson (seventy-five subs), and many parish churches (one or two subs per parish).

In 1911 it appears that there was an educational activity organised by the doctors as one of them, Dr Herepath, published a paper in the *Bristol Medico-Chirurgical Journal* on auricular fibrillation that stated was 'read before the Bristol Dispensary Clinical Society'.[43]

The Role of the Committee

The committee consisted of twelve men and a secretary and treasurer and were elected at the annual meetings from the subscribers. They were usually businessmen but there were a few doctors.

Table 8   Bristol Dispensary Committee Members

Committee members	Date of appointment	notes
Henry Daniel	1879	
Fenwick Richards	1879	
J Hudson Smith	1884	
S Day Wills	1884	
R Shingleton Smith	1885	physician at Infirmary, on committee for 44 years
J WStone Dix	1885	
Herbert Nash	1885	
H Addiscott	1899	
Herbert M Baker	1900	
James H Howell	1901	
Francis Sturge	1902	
Roderick J Fry	1903	
Thomas Davey	1904	
John Curle	1905	
Norman Wills	1906	
G Palliser Martin	1914	
TH Smith	1915	
Dr George Parker	1921	physician at General Hospital and former dispensary doctor
F N Colborne	1923	
Clifford Steadman	1923	
Arthur E Harris	1925	
Dr Leonard A Moore	1927	general practitioner and former dispensary doctor

Dr Kenneth Wills	1927	dermatologist at General Hospital
F F Clothier	1929	
A E Cater	1929	
E Brookhouse Richards	1931	
C Merrett Stocks	1934	

The dispensary committee was responsible for the financial state of the dispensary and for appointing the staff, including the medical officers, dispensers, midwives, and secretaries. They had to decide the geographical cover of the dispensary and how far midwives and doctors could travel to see patients in their homes. As we have seen already, they had to ensure that only poor patients were seen, and inevitably there were problems. On one occasion, a letter was received from WH Ridgeway of Merchants Street, who considered himself and his family slighted by inquiries made by Dr Powell as to his position in life, and he demanded a written apology. The committee, having made all necessary inquiries, decided he was not entitled to ask for any apology. Dr Powell was justified in making the inquiries, which were not of an offensive character.

The committee also had to decide how long a doctor was appointed to his dispensary job. In December 1921 they felt that they could not see their way to extending the time medical officers were employed beyond fifteen years, but in 1922, they agreed to extend Doctors Elliott, Bergin, Morris, and Dixon's terms for a further two years in view of their war service. The next year they again approved the four doctors, along with Dr Finzel, for up to twenty years. In 1927 they agreed that an upper age limit of 55 be introduced. In 1923 a Dr Evans was considered too young to be appointed at 22 years of age, but as the preferred doctor resigned the next year, Dr Evans was appointed.

In 1883 the chairman felt he had to explain about a paragraph in the annual report as it implied that some patients may not be seen in the dispensary. Apparently, Dr Davies, the health officer of the city, had asked that all cases of smallpox and typhus should be isolated, so the committee instructed the medical officers to immediately report to Dr Davies if they come across such cases. It seems that some months earlier, notes had been given to such patients, and this contributed to the spread of the diseases.

Controlling the Doctors

The medical officers were not easy to control. For instance, in March 1906, Dr Newman was living outside his district and stated that his residence in Wells Road was fifteen to sixteen minutes' walk from his house to Mill Lane Dispensary by way of the new road and Windmill Park. This was not acceptable to the committee, so he had to move to Coronation Road, Bedminster. Another surgeon, Dr Webb, whose district was Barton Hill, asked if he could take over the district about to be vacated by Dr Powell; the committee discovered that Dr Webb had moved his residence to Brunswick Square (outside his district) without their knowledge or sanction, and after an interview decided they would sanction him continuing to live in Brunswick Square, but they could not agree to him changing his district.

In February 1908 Dr Pinniger applied to be allowed to take on the post of curatorship of the museum of the General Hospital and was given permission. In May 1908 Dr Morris applied to be allowed to take the post of honorary pathologist to the Bristol Children's Hospital. He stated that the work would not in any way interfere with his dispensary duties, and the committee agreed for him to do this. Dr Bergin asked for permission to take the post of honorary skiagraphist (radiologist) and clinical photographer to the General Hospital, and the committee approved, subject to the work not interfering with his duties. Two years before this (May 1906), Dr Richardson applied for permission to take the post of medical officer to the Life and Health Insurance Co in Bristol – but this was refused. After one or two years the doctors could take on private patients, but they had to request permission. The doctors had to provide and pay for their replacements if they became unwell.

In the 1930s, some of the doctors were employing their assistants to do their dispensary work, and the committee objected. In March 1931 the secretary reported that Dr Dixon's work at the dispensary was being still being carried on by an assistant although some time previously Dr Dixon had given an assurance that he would give his personal attention to the work. The committee decided that the work of the institution must be given individual attention by each medical officer. The secretary was instructed to write to Dr Dixon and suggest he should submit his resignation. The next month Dr Dixon was reported as attending to his work at the dispensary.

In 1935 Dr Duerdon was also reported as not complying with the rules and was delegating his work to a partner and to his assistant, and he was persuaded to resign. Not only were patients not being seen by the medical officers, there was concern over delays in patients being seen at all. Patients were not to be kept waiting for two to three hours – dispensary patients should be given first attention.

The Doctors' Requests to the Committee

Drs Newman and Coleridge requested some new instruments for the Bedminster Dispensary, and this was agreed, at a cost of £6. It being a quarterly meeting, the medical staff joined the committee, and a request was made that they might have 'washing bowels (sic) in the consulting rooms', as well as testing glasses. The committee was pleased to grant the request.

The medical staff made application that they might occasionally have the use of a waiting room in the evening for purposes of consultation; such uses would be only three or four times in each year. The committee took pleasure in granting this request.[44] Dr Finzel requested that he could receive a non-monetary present from the friends and relations of a deceased patient, and this was agreed.

In 1932 a weighing machine was provided for each dispensary following a request by Dr Dixon. In 1936 Dr Morris stated that the staff had great difficulty in parking their cars near the dispensary and wondered if a building adjoining the dispensary could be used as a garage. This too was arranged.

The Financial State of the Dispensary in 1907

At the annual meeting,[45] it was reported that during the year, 9,847 patients were cured or relieved, 256 had died, and 1,306 remained on the admission books. Five hundred and sixty-two women were delivered, and 568 children were born. The cost of medicines was £432 7s 11d, and salaries and wages were £2,312 5s.

There was a considerable amount of income from investments (more than £2,000) and a few substantial legacies. It appears then that the dispensary was financially secure, and in 1910 the old North Road premises were sold for £750, primarily because it was becoming difficult to ensure that a rent could be collected. In 1908 it was decided to reduce the cost of becoming a life subscriber from £21 to £15.15s.

The National Insurance Act of 1911

This Act was introduced by the Asquith Liberal Government to provide for insurance against loss of health, for the prevention and cure of sickness, and for insurance against unemployment for waged earners, but not for their dependants and the unemployed. Voluntary charitable organisations like the dispensary were uncertain how this would affect their future. All workers who earned less than £160 a year had to pay 4d a week to the scheme; the employer paid 3d, and general taxation paid 2d (Lloyd George called it the 'nine pence for four pence'). As a result, workers could take sick leave and be paid 10 shillings a week for the first thirteen weeks and 5 shillings a week for the next thirteen weeks. Workers also gained access to free treatment for tuberculosis, and the sick were eligible for treatment by a panel doctor. The National Insurance Act also provided maternity benefits. At a special general meeting of the dispensary in 1914 the meeting approved the rule that midwifery notes would not be available for any woman whose husband was an insured person.

Before the Act was passed, the committee received a letter on 16 June 1910 from the Sunderland Provident Dispensary and the Tottenham and Edmonton General Dispensary stating that they thought the National Insurance Bill in its present state would seriously affect the subscription of all charitable institutions and asked if the Bristol Dispensary would consider if any concerted steps could be taken to get the provident dispensaries recognised in the insurance bill. The committee replied that they needed more information before committing themselves. Another letter was received from the Bristol Civic League on 15 September 1911 asking about cooperating in starting a dispensary for tuberculosis treatment. The committee replied that until they saw the effect of the National Insurance Bill on the subscriptions, it would not be appropriate to do this.

On 19 July 1912, the staff suggested the committee should alter the rules so as to exclude any insured persons under the Act obtaining relief by dispensary notes. At the annual meeting on 10 January 1913, Dr Shingleton Smith (committee member) said that in Bristol, the medical men had come to an agreement with the insurance committee. All the dispensary staff except one had placed their names on the panel and were ready to see insured persons, as well as others. The medical staff were now free to see patients whether insured or not. He said that very few insured people were likely to come to the dispensary when they had the choice of 120 doctors on the panel, whom they could see in the evenings after the dispensary and business hours. He pointed out that although the insured persons might be provided for, the women and children, who were about 80 per cent of their patients, were not, and therefore the need of the institution was as great as ever.

The committee stated that any patient who came with a note, whether insured or not, must be seen and attended to by the medical staff. In 1913 there were several complaints from patients on the very long time that they were kept waiting owing to the very late attendance of some of the medical staff. A letter was written to the medical officers about this.

Problems during World War 1

According to the annual report on 8 January 1915, there were nine medical men looking after more than ten thousand patients. Two of the medical officers (drs Herepath and Dixon) had volunteered and gone to the front, where they were doing good work. The duties of one of these men is being done by a colleague and the other by his father who was formerly on the staff of the dispensary. One of the members of the committee (Mr JS Davey) had been killed in action. He had been replaced by Mr TH Smith representing the Bristol Workers Medical Institute Fund, thus making the dispensary the first institution in the city to invite a representative of the employees to sit upon its committee.

In 1917 Dr Elliott reported that almost all the remainder of the medical staff had been called up. They had received six days' notice, which had subsequently been cancelled and a months' notice given, to expire on 19 May. The secretary reported that he had asked each medical officer to appeal and also sent them a covering letter to put before the medical board, stating that it would be impossible to carry on the work of the institution, five out of nine medical officers having already been taken. As many of the patients were wives and children of soldiers at the front, it was more than important that no further officers be called up.

However, Doctors Elliott and Robertson were both called up. Later, a letter was received from Dr Robertson, now a prisoner in Germany. He was well and had a private room for himself and sufficient food to eat. Dr Herepath had been decorated with the Military Cross.

In 1918 midwifery notes were now being subjected to an extra charge of 7/6 by the midwives. The secretary explained that the notes were originally free but the midwives now charged an extra five shillings per case, which they were now raising to 7/6. The reason they provided was that under the dispensary rules, the midwife attended the confinement, washed the baby, and paid four visits during ten days under the Central Midwifery Board, rules to which all midwives were attached. They had to visit each day for ten days, as well as pay a large amount of extra attention, which would be impossible for them to give at a fee of 7/6 – in their private cases, the charge was 17/6.

The Bristol Lying-In Institution, whose notes were originally free, now had printed on them a notice that each patient should be charged an extra 5 shillings, and it was very probable that this would be raised to 7/6. The committee decided that if the patient was in very poor circumstances and thought the note was free of any extra charge, then the institute would remit the midwife an extra 7/6 so the patient could be attended free.

Financial Difficulties in the 1920 and '30s

The salaries of the medical officers were increased to £350 per year in 1920, but this immediately caused financial difficulties. A year later (19 November 1920), a proposal was made to increase subscriptions from a guinea to £1 11 shillings and sixpence each, and rule 39 was amended, reducing the number of weeks a patient was entitled to medical attendance from six to four. The next year the committee suggested reducing the salaries to £300 per year in view of the adverse balance in the accounts, as they felt they could not continue to pay large salaries of £350 per annum.

There were increasing requests to extend the area that the dispensary covered, and in 1923, the committee agreed to add a tenth district to the east of the city, and in 1928 a new district in Bedminster was approved, with newly appointed medical officers. Requests continued as many poor people who had previously lived in poor parts of Bristol had been removed to houses in the suburbs.

In 1931 the number of patients attended by each member of the medical staff was examined. They regretted to see the low number of 53 attended by Dr Dixon in the Bedminster District. The highest was 1,408 in No 5 District by Dr Finzel. The committee thought Dr Dixon should be prepared to take a lesser salary and wrote him a letter indicating this, as it was not possible to increase the size of his district. Dr Dixon suggested a salary of £200, and this was agreed.

By 1933 the financial situation was worsening, with four hundred fewer subscriptions being received, and a proposal was put to the doctors that they should receive salaries related to the number of notes attended by each of them.

Table 9   Suggested salaries associated with numbers of notes received each year

Number of notes	Proposed salary
500-600	£200.00
600-700	£220.00
700-800	£240.00
800-900	£260.00
900-1000	£280.00
1000	£300.00

Not surprisingly, the medical officers opposed this proposal, and the committee then gave notice that they would terminate four appointments at the end of the year. But by December the committee decided to go ahead with the original proposal and, in addition, to remove one district. They also inserted advertisements in the local newspaper for more funds.

In 1937, 11,862 new patients were seen during the year, eight women delivered, and 2,160 notes were sold. The secretary reported that there was a big increase in the drug bill during that year, a considerable amount of which came from the Bedminster Dispensary. The accounts were examined and found that one of the reasons was that following the resignation of the dispenser who had been employed for nearly fifty years, shortages were discovered and needed to be replenished. Also, some of the medical officers prescribed very expensive medicines.

The annual report of 1938 reported that following the slum clearance schemes, which sent large numbers of poorer people into the Knowle new housing estate, it was necessary that a branch be opened there. Money would be required as the dispensary hadn't the investments to provide this.

How Was the Dispensary Viewed by the Rest of Bristol in the 1920s?

In an unidentified local newspaper report in January[46] 1927, the correspondent wrote:

> Castle Green is a thoroughfare little used by the general public, and other than people whose business takes them there it is probably only resorted to as a quiet cut to avoid the crowd in Castle Street. It is, therefore, no exaggeration to say that there must be some thousands of Bristolians who are unaware that in Castle Green there stands a rather austere building bearing the name 'Bristol Dispensary', while of those who have seen it many probably dismiss it from their minds with the thought, *A place where you get medicine, I suppose.* In a way, these people are right: it is a place where one obtains medicine, but of the all-important thing they are ignorant – it is one of the finest of the numerous charities Bristol possesses, for its clients are the poor. And it is also one of the least known of the Bristol charities, for it dispenses its charity in the form of free medical assistance and medicine quietly and unobtrusively, and publicity rarely comes its way.

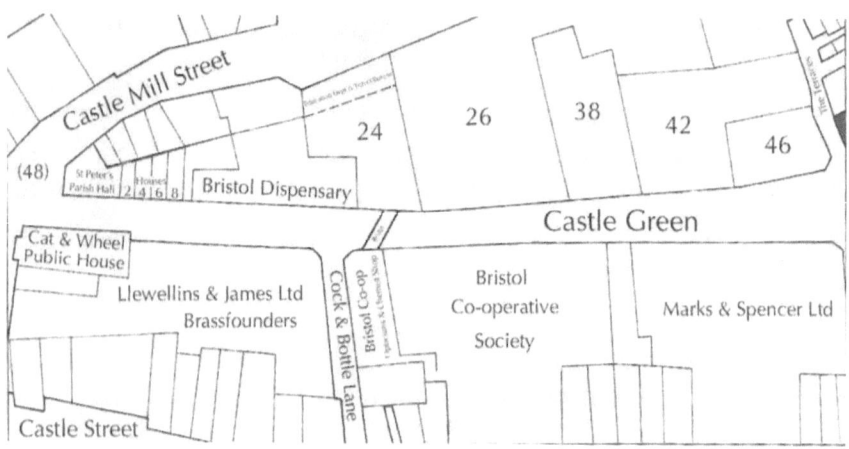

Map illustrating position of dispensary

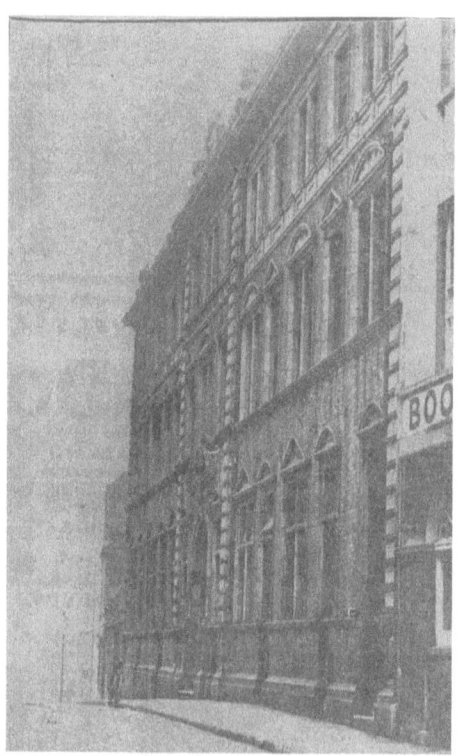

Image of the Bristol Dispensary from the 1929 minute
book of the dispensary in the Bristol Record Office
BRO 33041/BMC/13/3 (with permission)

The chairman of the committee in 1929, Norman Wills, stated that 'possibly someday, Bristol Dispensary would become the outpatient department of the big Bristol institutions, with the added advantage of visiting the homes of those unable to attend the dispensary'. Mr Wills wished to draw attention of subscribers to the fact that during the year, they'd had an increase in the number of those who had obtained notes but certainly did not belong to the class for whom the dispensary existed. He appealed to subscribers to take care to see that the patients were suitable, for dispensaries were not a medical club. In that year the dispensary had helped 12,708 patients, and only 59 women had had babies, as the call for midwifery care had fallen off over the previous few decades.

In January 1941 the committee decided that no annual meeting would be held that year as the building had been destroyed by enemy action on 24 November 1940. A certain quantity of medicines was recovered from the dispensary ruins, and in the course of a week, premises were taken in Dean Street, St Paul's. There, six doctors were available. Misfortune followed; the work had been in progress but a few days when that building was totally destroyed by a bomb. Thankfully, no lives were lost at either place. The doctors and staff were quickly able to carry on their good work at St Luke's Mission Hall, Barton Hill, owing to the kindness of the vicar, the Revd Beaven. The story of misfortune, however, had not ended, as the branch at Mill Lane, Bedminster, suffered badly – all windows were smashed, many doors destroyed, and a serious loss of medicines occurred.

After the Castle Green building was destroyed in 1940, the dispensary moved to premises loaned by the Guild of the Handicapped in Bragg's Lane, but the work of the dispensary ceased with the advent of the National Health Service in 1948, and the remaining funds were administered by the Bristol Municipal Charities.[47] The last annual report in 1947[48] stated that subscriptions remained at one and a half guineas each, with the patient having to pay three shillings and nine pence on presenting at the dispensary.

Many families were involved in the Bristol Dispensary over the years of its existence. This can be seen among committee members, with the Stock family as an incredible example. As Bruce Perry wrote in 1984,[49] 'Mr TCM Stock was preceded in the office [of clerk to the dispensary] by his great-grandfather, his grandfather, and his father, an extraordinary record of interest in and work for a charity by one family'. The Fry and Wills families on the committee and the Leonard and Finzel families as doctors also had at least two members of their families being associated with the dispensary over many years.

In 1939 Mr Wills revealed that with the election of Mr Anthony Steadman, there would be no fewer than three fathers and three sons – Norman and Ralph Wills; Clifford and Anthony Steadman; and H Merrett and C Merrett Stock – on the committee.

The doctors working for the dispensary were a very mixed set of men. Many did not become well-known names in Bristol, but one (Bruce Perry) subsequently became a professor of medicine, and at least two became physicians in Bristol hospitals (Keith Herepath at the Infirmary and George Parker at the General Hospital). Some developed large private practices, but most didn't.

Chapter 3

THE CLIFTON DISPENSARY

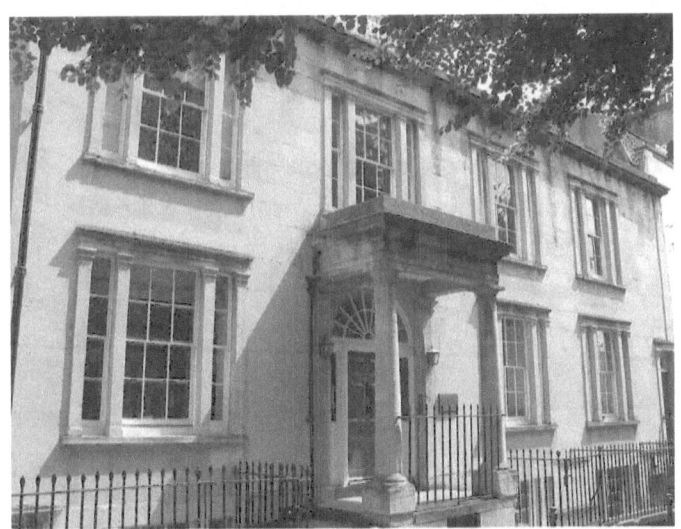

The Clifton Dispensary in Dowry Square 2009

Clifton is an inner-city suburb to the west of Bristol that was incorporated into Bristol in the 1830s. It contains the mostly affluent area of 'upper' Clifton, which was developed during the nineteenth century on the backs of the slave trade and tobacco industry, and the mostly poor area of Hotwells bordering the docks.

Dr Chisholm, a Clifton physician who was born in Scotland in 1755, suggested to a 'few respectable and benevolent inhabitants' the benefits that would arise from a dispensary in the parish of Clifton.[50]

On 29 October 1812, a meeting took place in the schoolroom to agree to establish a dispensary for the indigent sick in Clifton. Three months later, a general meeting took place to confirm the rules and regulations of the dispensary. These included the appointment of two committees – one of twelve gentlemen and one of twelve ladies who would meet monthly in the dispensary room. A treasurer and secretary were also appointed.

Neve[51] suggests that the supporters of the Clifton Dispensary wished to create a charity that improved on the performance of the late Thomas Beddoes's Preventive Medical Institution on the other side of the Square and on Broad Quay, but there is no evidence to support his thesis. The first annual meeting of the dispensary took place on 10 January 1814, and the vicar of Clifton, Revd J. Hensman, was chair.

The two physicians to the institution were Chisholm and James Cowles Prichard. Colin Chisholm was originally a military surgeon to the British forces in the American War of Independence. After the war was over, he moved to practise medicine in Grenada in 1783 and in 1790 purchased a cotton plantation. In 1793 he married and moved back to Bristol, where it was reported that he had a good medical practice. Chisholm was elected a fellow of the Royal Society on 24 November 1808. His latter days were mainly spent in retirement on the continent. He died in London at the beginning of 1825. In one of his publications he described the illnesses the dispensary doctors dealt with in the first four years (see table 10).

Table 10   Diseases seen in the Clifton Dispensary (from The Edinburgh Medical and Surgical Journal 1 July 1817

A TABLE of Diseases which occurred at the Clifton Dispensary, with the events of each,—from 1st January 1815, to 31st December 1816.

Diseases.	Cured.	Dead.	Diseases.	Cured.	Dead.
Amaurosis	1		Enteritis	48	3
Amenorrhœa	17		Epilepsia	13	
Abortus	4		Epistaxis	1	
Anasarca	19	2	Erysipelas	16	
Angina Pectoris	1		Erythema	20	
Anthrax	1	1	Elephantiasis	1	
Aphthæ	1		Febris intermit. infant.	3	
Apoplexia	6	5	—— catarrhalis	8	
Arthritis rheumat.	2		—— quotidiana	1	
—— podagra	4		Gastritis	6	
—— retrocedens	1	1	Gastrodynia	6	
Anthrodynia syphilit.	1		Gonorrhœa balani	1	
Ascites	8	6	Hæmatemesis	7	
Asthma	34	1	Hæmaturia	4	
Atrophia	32	6	Hæmorrhois	12	
Bronchocele	1		Hemiplegia	8	
Catarrhus chronic.	3		Hepatitis acuta	64	2
Catarrhus	21		—— typhoides	2	1
Catalepsis	2	1	—— chronica	46	1
Cancer uteri	3	3	—— gangrenosa	1	1
Cephalæa	22	1	—— apostematosa	1	
—— syphilitica	1		Hepatalgia calculosa	11	
—— ab ictu	2		Herpes	1	
Chorea sancti Viti	4		Hydrops pericardii	1	1
Cholera morbus	6		Hydrothorax	15	6
Convulsio	15		Hydroceph. acut.	37	8
Carditis	9	2	—— chronicus	1	
Constipatio	12		Hypochondriasis	5	
Contusio hypochond.	5		Hysteria	26	
Colica pictonum	2		—— cataloptica	4	
Cynanche laryngæa	1		—— hepatica	23	
—— stridula	4		Hysteritis	7	
—— parotidœa	2		Icterus	9	
—— tonsillaris	13		Ileus	1	
—— maligna	1		Lethargus	1	
—— syphilitica	2		Lepra	1	
Crapula	1		Lienteria	3	
Debilitas senilis	2		Leucorrhœa	10	
Dentitio	5		Lumbago	2	
Diarrhœa	14		Læsio uteri	1	1
Diabetes	2		Lichen	1	
Dysenteria	10		Marasmus	7	
Dyspepsia	6		Melæna	1	1

Diseases.	Cured.	Dead.	Diseases.	Cured.	Dead.
Melancholia religiosa	4		Scrofula vulgaris	51	2
Mania	1		Scarlatina	13	
Mastodynia	1		Scirrhus hepatis	1	1
Menorrhagia	15		Synochus	36	
Menses cessantes	25		Syncope	1	
Mollities ossium	1		Senilitas	3	1
Myocolitis	1		Scorbutus	1	
Nephritis	19		Splenitis	1	
Ophthalmia	5		—— apostematosa	1	
Paralysis	10	2	Strictura recti	1	1
Pertussis	18	2	Syphilis	2	
Peritonitis	4		Tabes nutricum	10	
Phrenitis	5		—— mesenterica	2	
Phthisis pulmonalis	84	23	Tænia	11	
—— pul. incip.	31		Tussis	34	
—— hepaticæ	1	1	Tinea capitis	2	
Pneumonia	188	2	Trismus dolorificus	1	
—— typhoides	6	1	Typhus	16	4
Prolapsus ani	1		Urticaria	2	
—— uteri	4	1	Variola	2	1
Psora	9		Vermes intest. lumb. ascarid.	90	
Pyrosis	5		Vertigo	9	
Proctalgia inflammat.	1		Miscellanea	55	
Psoriasis diffusa	10				
Rheumatismus acut.	76		Total Number 1699} or 1 in		
—— chronicus 28			Of whom died 101} about 17		
Rubeola	55	5			

James Cowles Prichard was also appointed as a physician to the dispensary for a year or two, having also been appointed physician to St Peter's Hospital in 1812, but he had started up his own dispensary for the poor when he arrived in Bristol in 1810 (see pages 5-7). Two surgeons, Peter de Jersey (who was to be the dispenser) and Mr Roblyn, were also on staff. There were 554 admissions in 1813, 160 of these receiving vaccinations.

Roblyn was born in 1779 and was a naval surgeon. He practised as a surgeon and physician in Clifton for many years after leaving the navy and in 1830 was living in Dove House, Dowry Square. In 1837, he was described as a physician and living in Cornwallis Crescent, Clifton. He was highly and deservedly respected, married Rebecca Rolls in 1835, and died in 1855 in Weston-super-Mare.

The report of the dispensary in 1813[52] states that the population of Clifton was 8,000 at this time; that 4,000 people were 'in a state of dependence or indigence'. There were 184 subscribers, and receipts and outlays were running at £191 in this first year. Activities in the second year increased slightly: a financial turnover of £240, with 487 cases dealt with, including 100 vaccinations.

All the major Clifton families figure into the list of subscribers. The dispensary was open for two hours a day, and the chronically sick were to present themselves, complete with recommendatory ticket, between ten and noon on Tuesdays and Fridays. Patients had to be residents of the parish of Clifton, and 'no person was to be considered an object of the institution who had not been a bona fide resident in the parish for at least three months'[53]. Rule XVII stated that 'no domestic servant whilst actually residing under his or her master's or mistress's roof would be deemed an object of the charity'. By the mid-1820s, the Clifton Dispensary was in financial difficulties, and the efficiency of its subscription system was failing. Despite a drive on parish collections, these yielded only £95.

The rules provided that patients of the institution had no other means of obtaining medical assistance at the time of admission. The institution was under the management of life members of £10.10s each and annual subscribers of a guinea each. Subscribers and donors were entitled to receive four sick notes and one midwifery note, or six sick notes. Additional tickets could be obtained at the dispensary at the rate of 4s for each sick note and 10s for each midwifery note.

The scale of activities at the dispensary increased slightly in the following years; the third annual report shows receipts and outlays of £226-11-5, with 683 cases seen in the previous year. The report states that one in every four of the 'indigent' of Clifton became 'objects' of the institution.

By 1820, the physicians increased to three: WH Gilby, DJH Dickson, and M Felix.

David James Dickson was a remarkable doctor who was appointed physician to the dispensary in 1817 to replace Chisholm.[54] Born in 1780, he became a surgeon's mate in the navy and in 1799 was promoted surgeon in 1800. In 1808 he was appointed physician, Leeward Islands Squadron, having obtained his MD from Aberdeen in 1806. He published several articles on fever. He transferred to London and was appointed physician to the Russian fleet in 1813. In 1814 he was appointed inspector of hospitals on the North American Station. He returned to England and moved to Clifton by 1816. He was admitted as a fellow of the Royal College of Physicians Edinburgh in 1816 and continued to publish papers on fever. He lived in The Mall in Clifton. Dickson then published a paper suggesting the advantage of a fever hospital in Clifton and Bristol.

Another medical journal commented on this article:[55]

'Dr Dickson's talents as an able physician and accurate pathologist, are already well known to his professional brethren. In this little pamphlet, distinguished by the classic purity of style, and the appropriate illustrations of its arguments, our author has embodied and compressed a great mass of evidence, tending to prove, not merely the utility, but the absolute necessity of houses of recovery in all the great towns of the kingdom. Those, therefore, who are about to propose or accelerate such laudable and humane measures, had better possess themselves of the pamphlet, and turn to their advantage the eloquence of our author'.

In 1824 Dickson was appointed physician at the Plymouth Naval Hospital and remained there until 1847. He was knighted in 1834 and died in 1850 in Plymouth.

Until 1822, the dispensary was situated in 1 Glocester Terrace, Hotwells, next to Granby Hill and just behind the Gloucester Hotel, moving to Dowry Square in 1823. The building in Dowry Square was erected and presented to the committee of the institution by Mr X by deed of trust dated 12 June 1823 and vested in a body of trustees, including Canon Hensman (the vicar of Clifton), Dr Howell (one of the Infirmary physicians), and Mr Durbin Brice.[56] In 1827 the duties of secretary and treasurer were filled by Mr Thomas Whippie, while the annual meeting was presided over by Admiral Sotheby. At that time the overseers of Clifton used to pay £35 for the care of the sick in the district, and the amount was afterwards increased to £50, but this grant was discontinued when the new Poor Law came into operation in 1837, the care of the paupers being transferred to an officer appointed by the board of guardians. In 1837 a legacy of £1,000 was received from the executors of the Mr Whippie, which was invested to provide meat, wine, and milk for those patients who the medical officers thought required this. In 1838 about a thousand patients received such sustenance.

The fifteenth annual report described a medical staff of two physicians and two surgeons, and that 1,752 sick cases had been dealt with for the year up to December 1827, but expenses were running at £436-6-9, with £60 payable to the apothecary Roblyn and £92 to Mr. Smerdon, the dispenser. Drugs cost £69-15-6, leaving a balance due to the treasurer of £57-3-6/d. It appears also that many applicants to the dispensary were refused service because of the inadequacy of their subscription tickets. The rules of the charity had been lightly altered, and vaccination was now offered without the need for a dispensary ticket; persons receiving parochial relief were also now entitled to tickets from the overseers of the parish. Debts continued with the shortfall in 1828 being £76-9s-4d. In 1829 the debt was somewhat reduced, and 839 cases seen, with 529 surgical, including ninety-one midwifery cases. In 1830 and 1831 an average of 800 medical cases and 450 surgical cases were seen. The report for 1832 shows the scale of activities increasing during the cholera epidemic when the poor could use the dispensary without any tickets, but at the recommendation of the Board of Health. There were 70 deaths from cholera recorded by the dispensary's medical staff. By 1839 the dispensary was used as a teaching site for those taking the exams of the Society of Apothecaries.

In 1828 John Howell was appointed physician to the dispensary after Gilby resigned. Like Chisholm, Dickson, and Roblyn, Howell had considerable military experience as a young man. He was born in 1777 and joined the army as a surgeon's mate in 1801, and became assistant surgeon in 1804 and surgeon to the Sicilian regiment in 1808. He was twice wounded in Egypt and in Portugal. He retired to Clifton and did excellent service during the cholera epidemic in 1832. He obtained his MRCS in 1801 and his Edinburgh MD in 1816. He was appointed physician to the Infirmary in 1829 until 1843. He died in 1857. He was looked upon as one of the leading physicians in Bristol.[57]

By 1830, the staff of the dispensary included the following physicians: M Felix, J Howell, Paris Dick; men-midwives T Roblyn and WJ Goodeve; and the dispenser, Mr Smerdon William James Goodeve was born in Hampshire in 1795 and in 1830 married Elizabeth Long Fox, who was the daughter of one of the physicians at the Infirmary and who had become the proprietor of one of the most famous asylums in Bristol, Brislington House. Unfortunately, Elizabeth died giving birth to their first child, and then Goodeve moved up the social scale by marrying Frances Erskine, the daughter of the Earl of Mar, with whom he had four children. She died in 1840.

Goodeve had trained in Bristol and had been assistant to Dr Gold, one of Bristol's earliest anatomy lecturers and took over these lecturers when Gold left Bristol. He failed to be appointed to the Infirmary on at least two occasions but was clearly a popular doctor as he was a member of the select Medical Reading Society of twelve members that had been formed in 1807.[58] In 1848 he remarried and had two more children. He died in Clifton in 1861 aged 66.

In 1833 there was an advertisement for an apothecary to the dispensary. The salary was £60 per annum with a house, and Samuel Oviett Goldney was appointed. He was a member of the well-known Goldney family of Cheltenham and Clifton. His younger brother was a solicitor and well-respected local politician involved in the Corporation of the Poor and was also on the gentlemen's committee of the dispensary. In 1839, Goldney, the apothecary, was declared bankrupt, and in 1841 he married the 16-year-old Caroline Rice, who unfortunately died the next year. The *London Gazette* in 1845[59] stated that 'Goldney was to be brought before the court for relief of insolvent debtors in Lincoln-Inn-Fields, London on 2 October 1845 to be dealt with according to the statute', and in the 1851 census, Goldney was described as health officer for Bristol City, but he died that same year.

Born in 1803, Gilbert Lyon was the son of a plantation owner in the West Indies and the holder of an Edinburgh MD. He had moved to Bristol in 1829 and was appointed physician to the Clifton Dispensary and to St Peter's Hospital in 1832. In 1839 he was delivering clinical lectures at the Clifton Dispensary to medical students. He resigned from St Peters when he was made physician at the Infirmary but retained his appointment at the dispensary until at least 1873.

Munro Smith[60] says of Lyon that, 'He had a large practice in Clifton and is still remembered by many as a clever physician, devoting great attention to the diet of his patients, which he was better qualified as he was, I am told, "an excellent cook"'.

In 1840 the honorary consulting physician was J Howell, and the physicians were G Lyon, W Kay, and W Trotman; the surgeons and men-midwives were T Roblyn and WJ Goodeve; and the apothecary was WD Wheeler.

William Trotman was born in Barbados in 1811 and was trained as a physician in Edinburgh. In 1845 he married Margaret, who was born in Bristol. They lived most of their time in Savile Row, Clifton.

Trotman was associated with the dispensary for more than thirty years.

Walter D Wheeler was born in Liverpool and spent some time working in Bristol at 23 College Green, when he was called an assistant surgeon, then at 11 Hanover Street. Before being appointed apothecary to the dispensary he was working at 65 Broad Quay in Bristol. In 1828 he was declared bankrupt.[61] There was clearly a problem in being an apothecary in Bristol at this time! However, despite having been declared bankrupt, Wheeler was appointed resident doctor at the Clifton Dispensary, and Wheeler and his wife, Sarah, had a one-year-old son in 1841. By 1851 the family moved to New York in the USA, where Wheeler worked as a physician.

In 1844 William Kay, the senior physician to the dispensary and lecturer on forensic medicine in the Bristol Medical School, was asked by the commissioners for the Health of Towns to write a report on Bristol and its vicinity.[62] This seventeen-page report on Clifton gives a very clear indication of the situation around the dispensary at the time.

Kay describes the medical record keeping at the dispensary set up at the suggestion of the medical officers. The headings for each patient were:

No. of Note
Date of admission
Patient's name
Age
single or married
Place of abode
Occupation
Disease
Physician consulted
Results (i.e., Relieved-Cured-Died)- Date
Observations -(Post mortem appearances, Etc).

He continued: 'This arrangement, and the regularity and care with which the entries are made, renders it at all times easy, by casual inspection, to ascertain the prevalence or absence of disease, epidemic or otherwise, in any part of the district. Such a register, in short, affords what I consider every medical institution in the kingdom ought to be capable of supplying a very valuable summary of medical statistics'.

Kay's conclusions were that Clifton was a decidedly healthy locality. The general mortality was less than most other towns with the exception of the metropolis. Infant mortality was least; more persons attained advanced ages, from fifty to seventy. Its two divisions, upper and lower, presented a marked contrast in almost every particular with considerable more than double the number of persons, in proportion to the population, dying *below* than *upon* the hill.

He finished by stating, 'Why should persons be allowed to erect human habitations, in situations and in construction, so palpably at variance with every principle of health or convenience? What right has any man to crowd human beings, poor thought they be, into a space utterly incompatible with wholesome, not to say comfortable, existence?'

In 1850 the honorary consulting physician was still Howell, and the physicians were GD Fripp, W Kay, and W Trotman; the surgeon and men-midwives were J Colthurst and WJ Goodeve; and the apothecary post was vacant.

Robert Watts, who was subsequently appointed apothecary, was born in 1802 in Bath and qualified LSA 1827 and MRCS in 1828. He was working as a locum at the Bristol Dispensary in Queen Square in the 1841 census and was appointed to the resident post at the Clifton Dispensary sometime before 1851. He remained in the post until he was 65 and then moved to London, dying in 1876.

Watts was involved in two court cases: Mary Smith was charged with obtaining a box of linen from the Clifton Dispensary under false pretences. She had presented herself pretending to be in labour, simulating so cleverly that she deceived two surgeons and the dispenser. She sold the linen at various places.[63] Then, in 1857, Watts gave evidence about a tallow maker who was producing a stench that had, he believed, caused forty to sixty cases of diarrhoea in the neighbourhood.[64]

GD Fripp was born in Bristol in 1805, the brother of physician James Fripp. In 1845 he obtained his MD from St Andrew's, and sometime before 1851 he left Bristol and started practising in London, initially in St Pancras and then in Regent's Park.

Colthurst was born in Bristol in 1811, the eldest son of a Bristol maltster. His medical education was initially in Bristol and then at St Bartholomew's Hospital, London. He followed this by training in large hospitals in Milan, Florence, and Naples, after which he taught Bristol students in practical and surgical anatomy from 1834 and then set up in practice in number 11 The Mall, Clifton. He was elected FRCS in 1844. He became a councillor for Clifton in 1854 and remained on the council until 1869. He was also active in other ways and was elected chairman of the gentleman's club, the subscription rooms (the Clifton Club) in the Mall for a number of years from 1858. He was appointed to Clifton College's foundation council in 1860. The 1861 census stated that he owned 257 acres in Somerset and also owned Chew Court, a mansion in Chew Magna. However, in 1867, having lost much money as a director of a railway company, he was declared bankrupt.

At the 1859 dispensary annual meeting, it was stated that Dr Kay had retired as physician and Dr John Beddoe has been appointed in his place. He retained this appointment for four years until he was appointed physician to the Infirmary. There had been 162 deliveries during the year, including two sets of twins and one of triplets. There were 2,110 successfully treated cases.

By 1870, the staff of the dispensary included physicians G Lyon, W Trotman, J Lancaster, and JG Swayne; surgeons T Sawyer, J Metford, and TGL Baretti; and resident medical officer JDT Parsons. Weekly notices in the local newspapers indicated which surgeon and physician would be on duty during the week.

Dr Joseph Lancaster, Mr Metford, and Mr Baretti were physician and surgeons respectively to the dispensary over about two decades. Lancaster was born in Clifton in 1811 and died in 1892. He was exceedingly well qualified with his membership of the Royal College of Physicians, the fellowship of the Royal College of Surgeons, and his MD from St Andrew's, but I could find no trace of any publication or appointment to any institution other than the Clifton Dispensary. He lived in very prestigious addresses, from Royal York Crescent to Cornwallis Crescent in Clifton.

Joseph Griffiths Swayne, born in 1819, obtained his London MD and was appointed lecturer in midwifery to the Bristol Medical School and achieved considerable fame as an obstetrician. In 1853 he was appointed physician-accoucheur to the newly opened General Hospital and retained his appointments for more than fifty years, ending as emeritus professor of midwifery. He published his well-known *Obstetric Aphorisms for the Use of Students* in 1856, which went to ten editions. His work was chiefly confined to outpatients, and he had no beds assigned to him in the hospital – any abdominal operations that were required were handed over to the surgeons. He became unwell and resigned his posts, travelling to New Zealand, but on his return to Bristol he was appointed initially to the post of physician to the dispensary but was then appointed to the more appropriate post of consulting accoucheur.

Born in 1825, Joseph Seymour Metford was the grandson of Joseph Metford a former surgeon to the Infirmary. In 1847 he gained the post of apothecary at the Infirmary and held that post for three years. After that he applied unsuccessfully for the surgeon's post at the Infirmary in 1854 and 1857. Metford was appointed honorary surgeon of the Clifton Dispensary and became interested in diseases of the ear. He set himself up as surgeon to a dispensary for diseases of the ear in Berkeley Crescent, Clifton, which lasted forty years. By 1871, he had moved, like his grandfather, to 31 Berkeley Square and was now calling himself a general practitioner. Finally, he moved to 34 West Mall Clifton before 1891 and died in 1895.

Thomas George L'enardi Baretti qualified in 1855 with the MRCS and LSA and was appointed surgeon to the dispensary in the late 1860s. He lived in Royal York Crescent and in the 1871 and 1881 censuses described himself as a general practitioner.

The resident medical officer (RMO), Dr John Dungate F Parsons, MD, had been the superintendent of the Whitehall House Asylum[65] in Fishponds from 1846. It shut down just before the Bristol Borough Asylum at Fishponds (Glenside Hospital) was opened in 1861. After the closure of the asylum, Parsons moved to the Clifton Dispensary in 1869. He died in 1886 at age seventy-two.

William Fyffe was a well-qualified physician with a military background. He was appointed physician to the Clifton Dispensary in 1873 but was not appointed as physician to the Bristol Royal Infirmary in a well-publicised election in 1876.[66] Fyffe died in 1901 in Clifton.

In 1878 the dispensary dealt with 2,164 medical, 231 surgical, and 172 midwifery cases,[67] and in the annual report of 1878, the following information about two charities available to the dispensary patients was described.

The Whippie Fund, which had been in existence for forty years and had been left 'to provide wine and meat to those recovering from the bed of sickness'. The fund was also useful for providing fresh air and change of scenery for many a patient at the convalescent home in Shirehampton. Later, it was mentioned that the Whippie Fund had been of great value to the sick poor; nearly four thousand pints of milk had been distributed, as well as brandy (nine quarts) and trusses supplied to all who needed them.

Mrs Lunnell's box charity provided valuable aid to the very poor women at their confinements by lending them an amply supplied box of linen for themselves and infants. In 1902 these necessaries were 'One and a half pounds of soap; 1 lb of oatmeal; 1 lb of sugar; tickets for 1cwt of coal and 1 and half pounds of meat'; and if the boxes were returned in good order, 'a set of baby linen'. Later, mothers were given '1s worth of eggs and 1 pint of milk a day for 10 days'. In 1908, seventy-two boxes were lent. In 1909, eighty-eight boxes; in 1914 it was sixty-four; from 1920–4 the average number was thirty-eight. The number decreased, until, in 1938, it was only two.

In the annual report of 1879,[68] it was stated that 'their total receipts are a little better than last year, though by no means commensurate with the wealth and growth of Clifton. There was a large expenditure for repairs in turning the basement from dark, cold and damp rooms, almost like cellars, into light, airy and cheerful ones, an alteration which the only wonder is that it had not been done years before'. At the AGM, one of the committee members noted that the provident element brought by the new half crown tickets being bought by patients at the Bristol Dispensary were proving useful; but it was decided that the Clifton Dispensary would not follow suit.

The weekly notice about the dispensary in the daily paper indicated that a degree of specialisation was creeping into the clinics. In 1890, for instance, diseases of the skin were seen on Mondays at 11 a.m.; diseases of the ear on Wednesdays at 10 a.m.; and diseases of women on Thursdays at 11 a.m. Other patients seen daily at 10 a.m. except Sundays. Both the Infirmary and the General Hospital were advertising special days for skin, ear, and women's problems at this time.

The year 1893 was a very busy one at the dispensary, with 4,871 cases being treated – an increase of nearly 1,500 over the previous year.[69] Almost half of the cases were emergencies (2,828); that is, they were treated without producing a note. There were only forty-five deaths reported – a reduction from sixty-seven the previous year. The chairman of the annual general meeting stated that the chapel and church collections for the dispensary were maintaining a downward tendency, being little more than half the amount that was given fifty years before when Clifton was little more than a fifth its present size. The resident medical officer was Thomas M Carter, a Bristol graduate, who remained in post for three years, being replaced by Mr W A Perry.

Very little information is available about the activities within the dispensary in the latter part of the nineteenth and early twentieth centuries, but the minute book from 1920 to 1940[70] gives details of the dispensary up to the second world war.

In 1920 there were 1,612 medical and 76 surgical admissions and the number of new notes was 1,443. There were 245 emergency cases, 3,209 visits to patient' houses, and 18 deaths. The number of patients showed an increase of 179 over those in 1919, and the number of visits to homes increased 814. The committee stated that the income at present was insufficient to carry on the work of the dispensary and to maintain the building in good condition. At the meeting, it was agreed to reduce the number of sick notes to life members and subscribers and donors of one guinea to five; of subscribers and donors of half a guinea to two sick notes and one child's note; and the charge for additional notes be 5s and for a child's note 2s 6d. Thanks were given to G Parker, MD; JE Shaw, MB; WC Swayne, MD; and LM Griffiths and RG Poole Lansdown, MD surgeons. The committee wanted to place on record their appreciation of Dr Dunn's services as resident medical officer. He was being paid £54 12s quarter. William Daniel Dunn was 77 years old in 1920 and was a retired doctor who had been running a practice in Nottingham before 'retiring' to Clifton.

Dr George Parker, one of the physicians, held a very special place in the history of the Bristol dispensaries. He was born in 1853 and took two Tripos examinations at Cambridge University, one in moral sciences and one in history, and then went to St Bartholomew's Hospital, London, qualifying MRCS and also took his MD. He moved to Bristol where he was appointed in 1887 to the Bristol Dispensary for five years before being appointed physician to the General Hospital. Parker was appointed to the committee of the Bristol Dispensary in 1921 and in 1918 was appointed honorary consulting physician to the Clifton Dispensary, having been serving on the committee of the dispensary for many years. He never married and lived in Pembroke Road, Clifton.

The chairman of the dispensary committee wrote in his obituary,[71] 'Although a busy man, he was one of the most regular members of our meetings, and was seldom absent. He took a keen interest in the work of the dispensary, and his advice was valued'.

In 1921, Doctors Lansdown and Shaw proposed that the committee should institute some scheme of contributory payment by those patients who could afford to do so, towards the cost of drugs and appliances. It was agreed to have notes divided into halves by perforations. A complete note entitled the patient to free treatment If only half a note was given, the patient would be required to pay 3s at the dispensary towards the cost of drugs and appliances before being accepted as a patient.

Dr Dunn resigned in December 1922, and Dr John Pollard, who had been acting as his locum, was appointed as resident medical officer. Apparently, this appointment was not a success, and in 1924, the committee decided to give Dr Pollard three months' notice and to appoint an RMO at a salary of £300 per annum, with a furnished house free of rates and tax and with lighting and coal. Accordingly, Dr Reginald George Francis Cookson was appointed RMO. It was arranged that midwifery cases were to be attended by qualified nurses from the Infirmary – the matron had to get permission from the BRI House Committee, and the cost of providing nurses from the Infirmary would be £100 per annum. The RMO requested that he might take private patients, and this was agreed, provided his private practice did not interfere with his duties at the dispensary, that his private patients were seen in his home and not the dispensary, and that the dispenser was not allowed to dispense any prescriptions for the RMO's private patients.

In 1925 the committee received a letter from the RMO stating that a patient, Mrs Maine, had been insolent and abusive and that he had refused to attend the case any longer. This was approved! The RMO inquired if the committee would pay the fees of a *locum tenens* (a fill-in doctor) while he was away on holiday. As it was not the practice for the committee to pay the fees of a locum tenens when the RMO had received permission to do private practice, and no exception was made in his case.

In 1926 Dr Cookson was provided with a steriliser at his request, and in 1927 he suggested alterations to the case books of the patients, stating he would like to keep a continuous record of their medical history. It was agreed to have these printed.

Chapter 4

THE OTHER BRISTOL DISPENSARIES

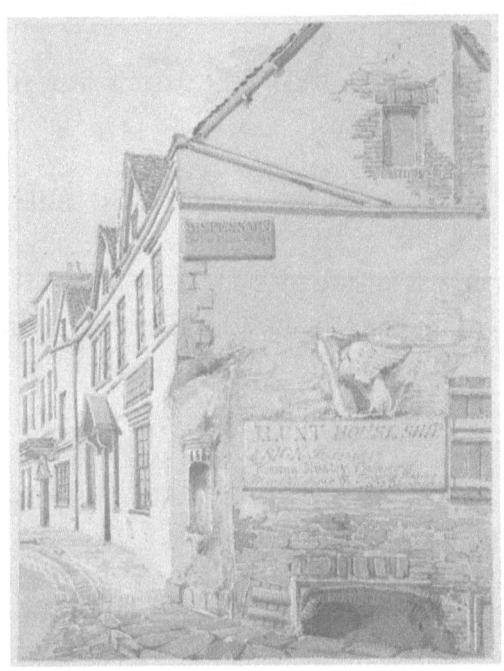

Bristol Eye Dispensary watercolour by Hugh O'Neill copyright
courtesy Bristol Museums, Galleries and Archives (M2548)

The Bristol Eye Dispensary

John Bishop Estlin was born in 1785, the son of the minister of the Lewins Mead Unitarian Church in Bristol, and was apprenticed to Mr Maurice, a neighbouring apothecary on St Michael's Hill, before undertaking an extensive education in Edinburgh, Paris, and Vienna. On his return to Bristol in 1808, he started practising from his home on Park Street. In 1811, he decided to open an eye dispensary in Frogmore Street to provide for poor patients without the need for them to get sponsorship from one of the subscribers to the Eye Hospital. He clearly shared James Prichard's views, which was perhaps not surprising since they were both members of an Edinburgh Medical Society, and Prichard was married to Estlin's younger sister. Estlin's dispensary lasted much longer than Prichard's and continued much beyond Estlin's death in 1855.

Estlin was prepared to work at the Bristol dispensary for a short time, as a newspaper notice dated 12 Sept 1812 states:

> 'At the dispensary lately established in castle green, a surgeon attends on Thursdays at one o'clock and on Sundays at nine to give advice to the poor'. There is written note[72] in Estlin's handwriting saying that the plan was suspended and saying that 'the notice about the dispensary in College Green was mine, but I resumed it again in Frogmore Street in September 1812'. Estlin continued attending his dispensary, and over the first thirty-two years of its existence, he worked alone and saw thirty-one thousand poor patients without charge, funding the first fifteen months running costs out of his own pocket. Patients attended there three mornings a week – Wednesdays, Fridays, and Sundays.[73]

Table 11   Activities at the Eye Dispensary

Year	No. admitted in year	No. subscribers	Other facts
1815	170	12	10 operations for cataract 20 corneal ulcers
1822	751		
1832	1374	84	

Each patient cost the dispensary one shilling. Each annual report of the eye dispensary gave detailed analysis of the conditions seen and treated. Estlin insisted that all who had not contracted smallpox should be vaccinated before being accepted for treatment at the eye dispensary.

Born in 1818, Augustin Prichard, James's second son, joined his uncle as surgeon at the eye dispensary. In 1850 he made his international name by being the first surgeon to remove a dead eye under chloroform anaesthesia to relieve the patient from severe eye pain and to save the sight of the other eye. In the same year he was elected surgeon to the Royal Infirmary. He continued to be associated with the Bristol Eye Dispensary, where he attended with great regularity, and, according to Munro Smith, 'did an enormous amount of useful work amongst the poor'.[74]

The number of patients admitted in 1856 was 2,205 and in 1857, 2,207 were seen. The dispensary was still open Wednesday at 1 p.m. and Sunday at 9 a.m. In 1860 Crosby Leonard was appointed assistant surgeon[75].

Two of Augustin Prichard's sons also became associated with the dispensary as surgeons. James Edward Prichard was born in 1849, and after spending time in Devon and south Wales in 1882 commenced private practice in Bristol. During his time in Bristol, he was connected with the eye dispensary on Orchard Street, to which he devoted much of his time, and where the loss of his skill and experience was much felt.

Arthur Prichard, born 1851, became consulting surgeon to the Royal Infirmary in 1906. For more than fifty years he was also in charge of the eye dispensary. In 1883 the dispensary was open on Sundays at 9 a.m. and Wednesdays at 1 p.m. Apparently, 116,029 patients had been seen since the dispensary opened, and fifty new cases were seen most weeks. The annual meeting in 1896[76] was described as 'the first upon its new basis' and followed the election of a management committee the previous year. A report had been received that indicated that structural alterations were required to the dispensary, new apparatus were required, and there was a need for more subscriptions.

Edgar Prichard, born 1861, Augustin's youngest son, was a solicitor and was present at this meeting.

Dispensary for the Cure of Diseases of the Eyes

Another eye dispensary was apparently started in 1890 in Merchants' Parade, Hotwell Road, when the surgeon Mr Henry Hetling was in attendance Mondays and Thursdays at 11 o'clock.[77]. Henry Hetling was the grandson of William Hetling, one of the Infirmary surgeons.

Bristol Vaccine Institution

John Bishop Estlin must also have been involved in starting this institution at 19 St Augustine's Place where 'attendance was given every Thursday morning at ten o'clock to vaccinate the children of the poor gratis. A deposit of sixpence will be required with each child, to be returned, if the child is brought again at the appointed time to have the arm examined. As Bristol and neighbourhood are seldom free from the smallpox, it is recommended that all children be vaccinated as soon as they are two months of age'.[78]

The surgeons JB Estlin, JC Swayne, WF Morgan, JG Wilson, GD Fripp, and WB Carpenter were all involved in the institute. The

Vaccine Institution was supported by voluntary contributions, and one of the surgeons attended in rotation for a month. The treasurer was Mr Estlin.[79]

Estlin appeared to have had a special interest in vaccination. In 1821 he circulated a questionnaire about vaccination to doctors in Bristol before giving a lecture on the subject. He asked

- How many cases of smallpox after vaccination have you seen?
- Did the smallpox go through its regular stages or was it in any respect modified either in duration or appearance
- Can you state how long the persons affected with smallpox had been vaccinated?
- In any of the cases, whether of modified or of regular smallpox, were there any doubts as to the vaccine disease having gone its usual course?
- Have you known any fatal case of smallpox after vaccination?
- Have you known any cases of smallpox occurring twice in the same individual; and, if so, was the secondary attack regular or modified?
- Have you known any case of this kind to be fatal?

The lecture was associated with a public meeting of the Philosophy and Literary Society and was held on 12 October 1821. The title of the paper was 'An Enquiry into the Value of Vaccination as a Preservative against Smallpox'.

In 1838 Estlin described the development of a new vaccine. He stated that he had been engaged in vaccinating for thirty years and had noticed a decline in the activity of the virus by the effect it was having on the skin of those vaccinated. He obtained a new source of vaccine from a cow in a Berkeley dairy and said the new vaccine was 'very energetic' and was now employed in many parts of England in preference to the lymph of the National Vaccine Institute.[80]

Bristol Institution for the Cure of Diseases of Children

In 1826 a dispensary for children, with the aim of benefiting the 'children of the industrious poor in Bristol and its vicinity by giving advice and medicine free of expense'[81] was created.

Attendance was daily at ten o'clock, and it was for the relief of every class of disease (with the exception of smallpox). A subscription was half a guinea a year. The treasurer was Thomas Bayly and the collector Mr Anthony. The consulting surgeon was Mr Daniel, and the surgeon was Frederic Granger.

Henry Daniel, born in 1783 in Bristol, was elected surgeon of the Infirmary in 1810. He married Cecilia James, and they initially lived at 16 Queen Square, moving later to Park Street. For some time he was in partnership with Frederic Granger, who previously was his pupil. Apparently, the profits were not great, and the partnership was ultimately dissolved in 1835.[82] Daniel had a good private practice and lived in some style, keeping a good carriage and fine pair of horses. He entered keenly into the social life of Bristol, was a notable Freemason, and devoted much of his leisure to botany and the cultivation of flowers and fruit. He died in 1836, and his daughter, Cecilia, married Infirmary physician Henry Riley.

Dr Granger was born in Bristol 30 January 1799 and decided against following his father as a hooper, as he disliked the trade. He was the second son. He became outdoor apprentice to Mr Daniel in 1820 and also paid thirty guineas to W Swayne as a perpetual pupil to the physicians. In 1820 there must have been some problem in getting his position with Mr Daniel, as his father, Mr Charles Granger, proposed to the trustees of the Infirmary that the existing rule that each surgeon should be restricted to three pupils or apprentices should be overturned. This proposal was rejected by sixty votes to thirty-five. Frederic then became a pupil at St Bartholomew's Hospital in London and qualified LSA in 1824 and MRCS in 1825. His first recorded address was 16 Park Street in 1830, and he soon after married Eliza Cooke at Queen Charlton.

In 1831 there was a notice that Fred Granger, MRCS, begged to announce to the medical students of Bristol that he intended to commence a course of lectures on the principles and practice of midwifery.[83]

Granger was consulting accoucheur to the Bristol Lying-In Institution, according to the 1831 annual report, and it was stated in that report that there had been 280 women delivered during the year (3,173 since the institution commenced). On the resignation of Henry Daniel from the Infirmary in 1836, he applied to become surgeon to the Infirmary but withdrew his application before the election took place. By 1851, he had moved to 22 Berkeley Square and died in 1886, having moved to Alveston Lodge on Durdham Down.

The Dispensary for Women and Children

In 1857 Mortimer Granville, the husband of Mary, one of Dr Henry Ormerod's sisters, opened a private dispensary for women and children at 17 Lower Castle Street. Henry became associated with it. In 1858 the institution moved to a house in St James Square. Dr Swayne was appointed honorary visiting physician; Mr W Ormerod (his father-in-law) honorary visiting surgeon, and Mr J Mortimer Granville and Mr H Ormerod honorary acting surgeons. In 1858 the dispensary moved to a house in St James Square, where it became known as The Free Institution for the treatment of diseases peculiar to Women and Children. Henry Ormerod and Mortimer Granville took turns being duty doctor to the institution for a week at a time. Attendances of patients were about ten women and between thirty and forty children a week.

In 1864 Mr Mark Whitwill, a Bristol merchant, visited Great Ormond Street Hospital, London, and decided to start a similar institution in Bristol. He received an invitation from the St James Square Dispensary to join their committee and realised that converting the dispensary into a hospital was a practical idea. Thus, the Bristol Children's Hospital was born, opening in 1866.

Unfortunately, Granville and his wife separated, and he went into practice in London.

Early in 1865, Mr Whitwill issued circulars to several personal friends, and these met with such a good response that later that year it was possible to acquire the house at number 7 Royal Fort Road.

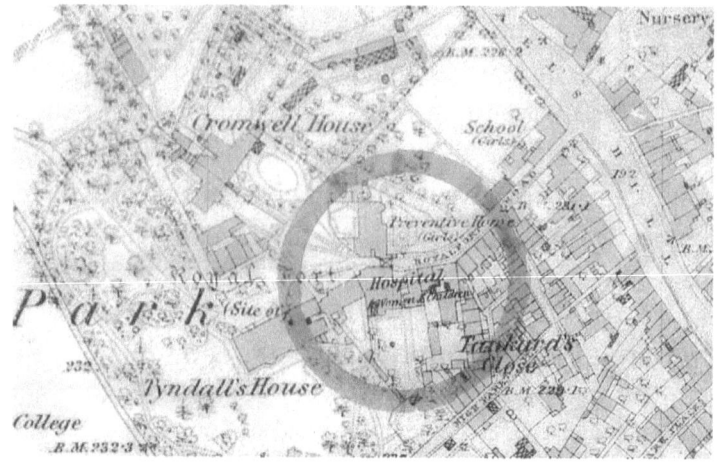

Site of Bristol Childrens' Dispensary. Map of Bristol (Ordinance Survey Sheet 1885 71.16 Gloucestershire)

To begin with, one room was fitted up with six beds; in the course of a few months, three more beds were added. On 25 October 1866, the first sick child was admitted into the institution. Between that date and 31 December, seventeen 'little sufferers were admitted to share in its benefits and blessings'.

It was designated The Bristol Hospital for Sick Children and for the Outdoor Treatment of Women, and its objects were

1. To provide for the reception, maintenance, and medical and surgical treatment of the children of the poor under ten years during sickness in a light and airy building, salubriously placed; to furnish with advice and medicine those who cannot or need not be admitted into the hospital. And also to receive as outpatients women suffering from diseases peculiar to their sex.

2. To promote the advancement of medical science with reference to the diseases of women and children and especially to provide for the instruction of students in these essential departments of medical knowledge.

3. To diffuse among all classes of the community and particularly among the poor, a better acquaintance with the management of infants and children during health and sickness, and to assist in the education and training of women in the special duties of Christian nurses.

The committee consisted of Earl Ducie (patron); Mr Whitwill (treasurer); Dr WG Carter (secretary); and the honorary medical officers Dr JA Symonds, Dr J.Beddoe, Mr C Greig, and Mr W Ormerod.

In 1858, at the first annual meeting of the Free Institution, Eubulus Williams was appointed assistant medical officer. He continued as a surgeon until 1862 when he resigned as a result of pressure from his private practice,[84] but at the repeated requests of one of the staff, he resumed his job. During the next few years, several other doctors started working for the Free Institution in St James Square: Dr Henderson as honorary physician, and W G Carter, G T Baretti, James McDonald, and Charles Steele as surgeons.

Dr Henderson, born 1825, who held the MRCP and MD, married Hester in 1853. They lived in Richmond Hill, Clifton, and had three children. In 1863 the marriage ended in an acrimonious divorce after Henderson left for America with another woman.

Thomas Baretti, born 1834 in Bath, lived in Royal York Crescent. He replaced Henry Ormerod and subsequently became a surgeon to the Clifton Dispensary. William Grover Carter was born in Guernsey in 1817 and lived in Bellevue, Clifton, and held the MRCP. In 1863, he resigned as a surgeon to the institution and was appointed physician. He had a very long association with the hospital, becoming secretary in 1866. James McDonald, born 1821, was appointed in 1863 and died in 1866 and had his practice in High Kingsdown.

Charles Steele[85] achieved FRCS in 1869 and obtained his MD in 1880. Born in Macclesfield, he studied at the Bristol Medical School and at the Bristol Royal Infirmary. He became surgeon to the Royal Infirmary in 1870 and lectured on physiology at the medical school. He was district medical officer for Clifton. He was for a time secretary and then member of council of the Bath and Bristol branch of the British Medical Association. He built up a large practice, both general and as a consultant, retiring from the Infirmary about 1908. He died, after a long illness, at Clifton Villa, on 20 September 1914. He was the introducer or inventor of a 'perfected clinical thermometer', of flexible probes, of chair supports for spinal curvature, and of steel spring splints.

At the special general meeting of subscribers and donors that was held in the new hospital on 25 August 1866, Mark Whitwill was the chairman and Dr Carter was the honorary secretary. The chairman said the new premises had plenty of fresh air and light; it was a house adapted for the purpose of an infant institution, and a nice piece of land was attached to it. There would be no noise, and £300 was needed to pay for the premises. The house was number 9 at the Royal Fort on the left-hand side at the top of Royal Fort Road.

The first patient was admitted on 26 October, and there was only one room with nine cots. In December 1867 there were 19 children inpatients. During the previous week 76 women had been seen in outpatients and 131 children.

Expansion took place quickly. By 1868 there were four wards with twenty-four beds; next year a bronchial ward was added, making thirty beds. In 1871, there were forty beds. In 1873, an infectious ward was added, and in 1876, a room was added for women needing an operation, who were expected to pay eight shillings a week. The present large site was bought in 1881.

One of the first woman doctors, Eliza Walker, who had obtained her MD at Zurich in 1873, competed with twelve male applicants for the position of resident medical officer at the Bristol Hospital for Sick Children. The medical staff objected to her appointment on the basis that she was unregistered – unavoidably so at the time.

However, the hospital committee 'were unanimously of the opinion that considering the special character of the institution as a hospital for children and a dispensary for women, there would be a peculiar fitness in electing a lady to the vacant office'.

Apparently aware that such a decision would incur the wrath of the hospital doctors, the committee called a special meeting of the subscribers, where the principle that medical doctors and nurses at the hospitals and surgical appointments should be open to women was upheld by a vote of seventy-two to seventeen. Walker was duly elected, and two of the consulting surgeons promptly resigned.

A month later one of the honorary staff also saw fit to resign over a 'misunderstanding' with Dr Walker and all the rest of the medical staff, but one, followed suit. Under these circumstances, within a few weeks, the resident medical officer felt obliged to tender her own resignation 'under terms which left [the committee members] no alternative but to accept it'. They may have heaved a collective sigh of relief, for the mass resignations had attracted much public attention, apart from being totally disruptive to the workings of the hospital. Eliza Walker changed her name to Eliza Walker Dunbar and continued to live in Bristol. She became medical officer for the Dispensary for Women and Children in Berkeley Square, Clifton.

General Dispensary for Children, Olivet Place, Redland

This other children's dispensary was advertised in 1870. It doesn't appear to have lasted long and appears to have been created to gain patients for Dr Webster, who lived nearby. The advertisement stated: 'This institution offers gratuitous advice and medicine to the poor on presenting a subscriber's note. Days of attendance: Monday, Wednesday, and Friday at half past ten. Medical attendants Mr Webster and Dr Daubeny'.[86]

Dr Thomas Webster was born in Ireland in 1818. He married Joseph Metford's daughter, Louise, in 1852. They had four children, none of whom married, and they all lived in a large house in Malvern

House in Redland Hill. Webster, having married into the Metford family, would have been able to compare notes with his brother-in-law, Joseph Seymour Metford, who was associated with the Institute for the Cure of Deafness and Diseases of the Ear.

Bristol Lying-In Institution

This institution was formed by William D Rolfe, one of the first doctors involved in the Bristol Dispensary, who became the first secretary of the institution. It was started in 1821 and the original notice stated[87]:

> The above institution has been formed for the *immediate* assistance of poor lying-in women either inhabitants of this city or casual poor, whose situation will not allow of the delay for the necessary form of admittance by the committee of the dispensary.
>
> That fatal consequences not infrequently result to mothers and children from the want of suitable aid is notorious. It is therefore an essential rule of this institution to employ only such midwives as are known to be duly qualified, and it is the constant care of the committee to watch over their conduct in every particular. Five shillings and upwards per annum constitutes a subscriber. For each five shillings two persons will be admitted.

The patroness was the Duchess Dowager of Beaufort; the treasurer was George Thorne. The physician was Matthias Felix, and the consultant accoucheur was Rolfe. The surgeons were Peter Challacombe and John Moss Chandler. In the first year 154 women were delivered.

The 1829 annual report stated that only married women were accepted and that, like the dispensary, a 'committee of ladies was annually appointed who meet monthly to regulate the affairs of the institution'. One of them in succession became the *visitor,* whose duty was to visit the poor lying-in women and afford them assistance so far as their limited funds would allow. A subscriber was now expected to contribute seven shillings a year, and 289 women were delivered that year.

William Dimmock Rolfe (1774–1831) left many of his books and Freemasonry regalia to his friend Richard Smith, who was a popular surgeon at the Infirmary. Rolfe did not make much money, and there is a note in Richard Smith's scrapbook from a fellow Freemason stating, 'I am much concerned to inform you that Miss Rolfe, daughter of our late brother and friend, WD Rolfe, died yesterday morning and much regret to add that the family are in such a destitute state that they have not a shilling to bury her. May I request on their behalf a trifle from your bounty that the poor girl may be interred in a decent manner?'[88] Richard Smith sent a guinea.

The Poor Lying-in Institution continued working for the rest of the nineteenth century.

The Bristol directories indicate that in 1845, the surgeons were EJ Staples, W James, and G Rogers, and a subscription still was seven shillings. In 1860 the surgeons were JG Swayne and Crosby Leonard, and in 1900 a subscription of £1 entitled the subscriber to four tickets of recommendation with Doctors H Cook and Chalmers Norton, the surgeons. The number of cases in 1897 was 270. The comment was added that this institute did not train midwives.

The Dispensary for the Care of Diseases of the Skin

This was sited at 3 Parade, St James's and was in existence before 1846 when the honorary physician was Dr James Fogo Bernard and the medical officer was Robert T H Bartley. This was the beginning of Bartley's professional relationship with the Bernard brothers (he was later to work with Ralph Bernard at the Eye Hospital). In 1853 he was in attendance at this dispensary from 11 until noon on Tuesdays.[89] Bartley appeared to be doing everything he could in order to get that elusive hospital appointment. In 1846 he published three papers in *The Lancet*. They were all on skin diseases and written from the Bristol Dispensary for Diseases of the Skin.[90] The first paper was about psoriasis and pityrisasis and the various treatments that Bartley had prescribed; the second was about impetigo of the scalp.

Towards the end of this second paper Bartley states:

> 'Of the cases applying for relief at the dispensary, at least three-eighths are children from the age of seven months to two years. This is to be accounted for from the fact that a large number of skin diseases at this early period are connected with the process of dentition, as well as with the susceptible condition of the mucous membrane of the stomach and bowels.... When the bowels are relaxed, of bad colour, and offensive, small doses of mercury with chalk, combined with rhubarb, I find most serviceable'.

Other remedies are described, including lancing the gums. The third paper in *The Lancet* was about eczema of the scalp and its treatment.

Another dispensary with the same title opened in 1885 under the care of John Hancocke Wathen (1845–1906) in Park Row and closed in 1895. Dr Wathen was an original member of the Dermatological Society of Great Britain and Ireland in 1894, and in 1898 presented his own experience of a local contact dermatitis due to iodoform gauze.[91] He was educated privately and at University College, London, and represented Clifton Ward on the Bristol City Council from 1893–96, becoming an Alderman in 1897.

Bristol Institute for Skin and General Diseases

This was originally opened as a dispensary in 1883 by Dr John Broom and was situated in 21 Nicholas Street, moving to 6 Colston Street until 1893, when it was moved to 13a College Green.

Patients were seen and treated for general diseases Mondays and Wednesdays 3 to 5 p.m.; Fridays 6 to 8 p.m. For skin diseases, hours were Tuesdays 6 to 8 p.m. and Thursdays and Saturdays ten to noon.

Patients were admitted for one months' free treatment (at the institution) on presenting a donor's or subscriber's admission note; they were also admitted on their own application and received treatment paying to the institution monthly, weekly, or casual contribution fees during the period of attendance.

The dispensary closed in 1900 on the occasion of Dr Broom's death. Dr Broom was trained at Durham and moved to Bristol from Sheffield, where he had a busy practice. He held the MD from Brussels with distinction. He married Eliza Sayles in 1873, they lived in Lancaster Villa, Clifton, and he became a partner of Dr Thomas Edward Clarke. However, this partnership was dissolved in 1879. It looks as if Dr Broom ran this dispensary on his own.

Bristol Provident Medical Institute

In 1876 a letter was received by the staff of the Infirmary from the Bristol and Clifton Charity Organisation Society inviting a representative of the faculty to attend a meeting to promote the establishment of provident dispensaries in Bristol.[92]

In 1883 John Lavars reported in the *Western Daily Post* that the Bristol Medical Institute occupied a space between the great charities and the private practice of the doctors. It worked on a principle that has long been accepted in several large towns. In Bristol, a committee of gentlemen took the lead and looked to the working classes to take advantage of the opportunity they put before them.

When, two years earlier, the Infirmary committee were compelled to make a special appeal to their supporters for help, it was prominently put forward that the vast number of outpatients to be admitted was one great cause of their difficulties. It was added that many of the persons relieved were such as ought to be above applying to a public charity, and were quite capable, with a little forethought, of making provision for paying for medical assistance in slight attacks of illness. This was not a difficulty of late growth with charitable institutions, as their real efficiency had long been crippled by claims for help with an ever-increasing multitude. Subscribers too often give away notes without sufficient inquiry into the circumstances of applicants, so that many of the working class and even those in better position are relieved from the necessity of making proper provision against sickness and are led into habits of dependence unhappily too common.

Looking round for a remedy for such a state of things, the originators of this institution considered that it would be best found in an arrangement by which the recipients of relief might themselves pay a regular subscription, by right of which they could demand assistance in times of need, and obtain it without feeling in need of charity. A committee had been formed in 1881 for this purpose, but the first decisive step in the formation of the institution was taken early in November 1882, when a meeting was held under the presidency of Dr Beddoe.

The committee met many times to inquire into the workings of similar institutions in other places and to decide on the best system to be adopted in Bristol. Several dispensaries in different parts of the city were already fitted up and doing good work in the hands of a private person, so it was determined to purchase and combine them under efficient and responsible management instead of establishing new ones, which would rival the old, to the injury perhaps of both. The purchase at a valuation was concluded, and at the beginning of the present year, five dispensaries were in working order, properly fitted with all necessary drugs and appliances, with duly qualified medical officers in attendance.

There was equal need with this institution as with charitable institutions for careful scrutiny, lest people who could well afford to pay the usual fees of a doctor should obtain admission to the injury of deserving members, and more so of the medical men whose great liberality in assisting the really needy would make the committee particularly careful in guarding their professional interests. From the first it was determined that the undertaking must be carried on a thoroughly businesslike basis and made self-supporting. It must not be a charitable institution but such as would appeal to the spirit of independence and thrift among those able to help themselves, and encourage them rather to rely on themselves for payment of their doctors' bills – as too many were in the habit of doing – on their rich neighbours. The thriftier among working men provided for times of sickness by becoming members of benefit societies or similar clubs.

It was probably more important to the poor than to the rich to have their ailments promptly attended to. Their bread depended on their health, and to be able to get a doctor at once often saved many a day's work to a poor man. Under the rules of this institution, patients not only could choose their own doctor from the staff, but they were visited by him at their own homes.

The five dispensaries now at work were situated in York St (St Paul's), Barton Hill, Easton, Hotwells, and Bedminster. Properly qualified doctors were only appointed and they attend each weekday at their several district dispensaries to see all members who presented themselves. Prescriptions were dispensed at the same place to avoid all delay and confusion, the necessary medicine being supplied free of cost. The expenses of working were met by members paying a small entrance fee and afterwards weekly sums of one penny for each adult, one and a half pence for a parent with one or two children, and two pence for larger families. Anyone joining when already sick paid in addition a fee of half a crown to cover the immediate demand on the funds. A proportion of the fee was handed periodically to the medical officers, and the remainder was applied to the purchase of drugs and to general expenses.

The attendances of patients from 1 Feb to the end of September 1883 amounted to 17,916 at the dispensaries and 2,427 at home. In Matthews Directory of 1900, the following dispensaries were still functioning: 129 Hotwells Road, Hotwells, Barton Hill, St Phillips; 177 Cheltenham Road, and 35 East Street, Bedminster.

It is interesting to compare this development with that of the Metropolitan Provident Medical Association. This was founded 'to relieve hospital abuse by means of forming providential dispensaries throughout the metropolis'.[93]

The Tottenham branch started about 1887, and ten years later it was found that about 16 per cent of members left the association annually, and 57 per cent of the membership were children 5 years of age and younger and their mothers between the ages of 20 and 40. Each member was seen on average 5.25 times a year, and severe illness was rare. The author concludes that provident association fails to relieve the mischief of the 'hospital loafer' and that unless some system can be created to obtain regular subscription throughout life and not just at critical periods such as surrounding childbirth and treating young children, they will not be able to compete with free hospital treatment.

Munro Smith included the following paragraph in his history of the Royal Infirmary[94]:

> In 1900 a suggestion was sent to the BRI Committee by the Christian Social Union that Provident Dispensaries should be established by the Infirmary and the General Hospital; that ordinary outpatients should be attended – these by dispensary doctors – and that the outpatient departments of the two medical charities (the Bristol Dispensary and the Clifton Dispensary) should be retained entirely for consultation cases to be sent by the dispensary medical officers, when necessary.

He added that this was not seriously considered at the time, but the idea in 1914 would no doubt be met with some support.

Forester's Medical Institute

The Friendly Societies developed in the middle of the eighteenth century, and the Ancient Order of Foresters was one of the largest of these in Bristol. The Friendly Societies were not just benefit societies. They were self-administered clubs that provided mutual insurance to members against sickness and death. All members paid a regular contribution, which gave them an agreed-upon entitlement to benefit if they were too ill to work.

The Royal Commission in 1874 on the Friendly Societies showed thirty-four existed in the United Kingdom, with more than a thousand members each.

They rapidly developed and grew in response to industrialisation, with 76,990 members in 1845 growing to 491,196 in 1875.[95] In 1887 the Bristol District of the Foresters contained 13,774 members in all, consisting of 11,677 financial members, 312 honorary members, 413 contributing widows, and 1372 juvenile members. The annual contributions were £15,144 to the sick and funeral fund, £528 for the subsidiary benefit funds, and £1816 to the medical aid fund. The expenditure of the three funds were £14,665; £457; and £1841 respectively, with about £74,000 in reserves.[96]

Most Friendly Societies employed their surgeons or medical officers on a contract basis to attend any member in sickness and to supply medicines in exchange for a payment of so much per member per year. A typical arrangement was:

> A surgeon shall be elected who shall continue in office during the pleasure of the court. It shall be his duty to examine all candidates; attend the sick members residing within three miles of the courthouse; and provide them with proper and sufficient medicine during their afflictions. The surgeon shall receive for each financial member ... 1s 6d per half year for his services.[97]

In 1870, starting in Preston, Friendly Societies developed medical institutes where doctors were hired full-time to look after their members. These institutes offered certain market advantages to the doctors. They had a regular income, and payment was guaranteed. But the capitation fees were low, and many doctors disliked the subordinate relationship the situation created.[98] At the beginning of the twentieth century, the relationship between the British Medical Association and the Friendly Societies deteriorated, and the 'contract system' that had developed between the Friendly Societies and the doctors gave way under the National Assistance Act of 1911, to the 'panel system', where the doctors were no longer under the control of Friendly Societies and hence their patients; they were simply consulted by their patients, thus re-establishing the typical doctor-patient relationship.

There is a Bristol newspaper report in 1874 about the destruction of the Foresters Music Hall (formerly the Alhambra) in Broadmead. Apparently, in June 1873 it had been purchased on behalf of the Bristol District of the Ancient Order of Foresters with the 'intention of converting it into a Foresters hall and dispensary, but the portion of the scheme relating to the formation of a dispensary had not been carried out'.[99]

In 1883, during one of the quarterly meetings of the society, one of the members proposed a toast to the Forester's Medical Institute and bore testimony to the skill of the medical staff and of the dispenser. The two were Dr Parette and Dr Ewens.[100]

Dr James Parette, born in 1846 in Paris was, despite his age, the senior of the two and died in 1885.

Dr John Ewens was born in 1830 in Axminster and trained at St George's Hospital, London. He practised in Cerne Abbas, Dorset, for about twenty-five years and then moved to Bristol, where in 1876 he obtained the job of surgeon to the Children's Hospital and also the second doctor to the Forester's Institute. He was especially interested in orthopaedic surgery, particularly in deformities of the foot.[101] He died in 1916.

In 1910 the institute was situated at 14 St James Square, and a clinic was held at 8 Russell Terrace, Dean Lane, Bedminster. The surgeons' hours of attendance were 9 to 11 a.m. and 6 to 8 p.m. The senior surgeon was Dr T A Collinson, who worked originally for the RAMC, and the junior surgeon was Dr L Hill Hay.[102] Dr Hay was a young Argentinean doctor who had qualified in Aberdeen and was working in Swindon in 1911.

Bristol Medical Mission

In 1871, at a meeting in the Victoria Rooms, Clifton, it was agreed to start medical mission work in Bristol. The key originator of this was Mr Benjamin Thomas, who remained the treasurer for more than twenty years. A building was found 'in the midst of a densely populated part of the city, and abounding with the class of people the mission hoped to benefit'. Redcross Street was just north of Old Market. The committee found considerable difficulty in finding a man who felt able to 'give their life to the double function of healing the sick and preaching the Gospel',[103] but eventually Dr Fountain Elwin FRCS was appointed and served the mission for about twenty-five years. He was educated at the Middlesex Hospital where he was clinical clerk and house surgeon, and at University College, London. He was at one time surgeon to the St George's and St James's Dispensary in London before moving to Bristol. He and his family lived on Clyde Road, Redland.

The mission was open without charge or fee to all poor persons on Mondays, Wednesdays, and Fridays at 10 a.m.

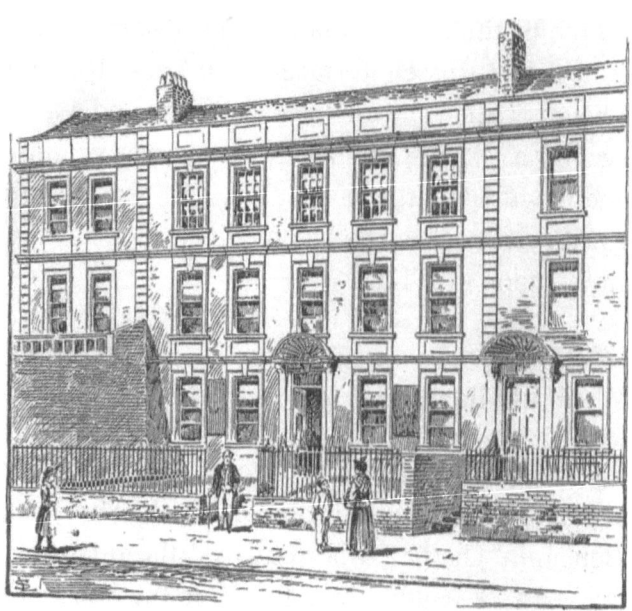

Bristol Medical Mission 7 Redcross Street
Courtesy of Bristol Reference Library

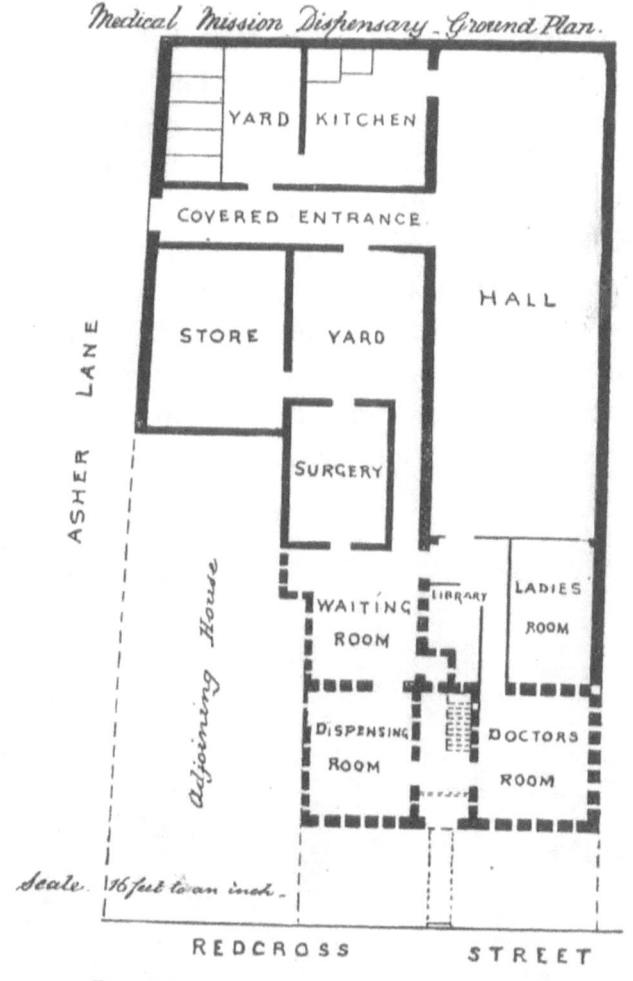

Plan of Medical Mission

The original dispensary is outlined in the hatched-lines,
the back of the premises was only developed in 1892. The
work of the mission changed considerably over time.

The clients included widows with large families, out-of-work
breadwinners, women and girls engaged in factories on scanty wages,
strangers to the city who came for work, deserted wives, and many
who sank low on the social scale. The mission work was confined to

the poor who were unable to pay for advice or medicine but weren't so poor as to be in constant need of parochial relief.

In 1877 a branch dispensary was opened at Barton Hill. This was served by Dr Kendall two days a week. Dr Sewell McFarlane was appointed successor to Dr Elwin and was helped by a dispenser, Dr Elwin having preferred to do the dispensing himself. McFarlane went to China to join the mission field in 1886 and was replaced by Dr William Elder, who had been serving as a missionary in India.

The mission was unable to retain the dispenser for financial reasons, so Dr Elder decided to instruct laywomen in chemistry, pharmacy, dispensing, and the care of the sick. Most of the forty-five he trained gained certificates and medals of the St John Ambulance Association.

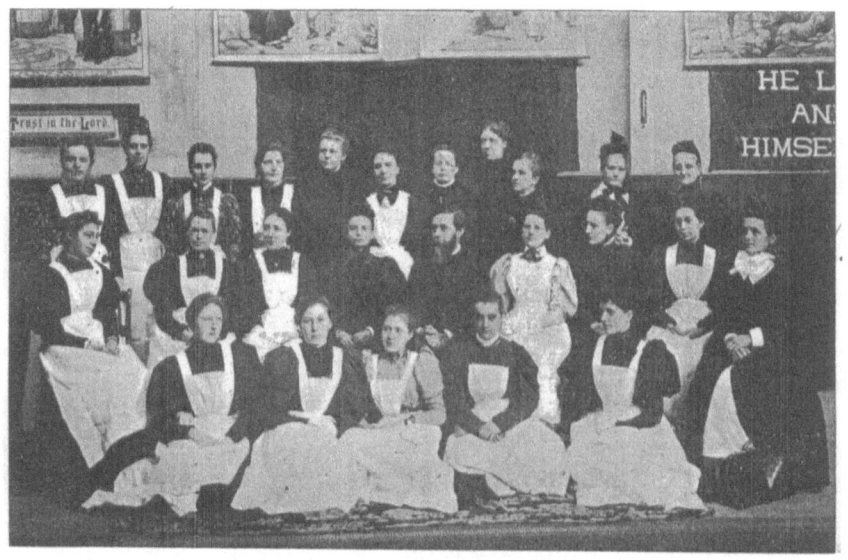

Dr Elder and the Mission staff. Photo courtesy
of Bristol Reference Library.

The medical superintendents were supported by two of Bristol's best known physicians, Dr E Long Fox, the senior physician at the Infirmary and by Dr W Johnstone Fyffe.

In 1873 the number of new patients was 1,609, and the attendances 6,724. In 1892, the number of new patients was 6,249, and the number of attendances 22,578. The 6,249 patients included 940 men, 3,985 women, and 1,324 children.

Their illnesses were:

Respiratory affections	2,066
Digestive disorders	1,361
Skin diseases	663
Rheumatism	397
Diseases of nervous system	105
Anaemia	94
Diseases of ear	72
Diseases of eye	65
Diseases of circulation	40
Vermes (worms)	21
Other diseases	465
Total	6,249

Home visits formed a considerable part of the work. Seven hundred thirty-two patients were seen at home in the one year: 85 men, 368 women, and 279 children. The description of one of these visits illustrates the home situations of many patients: One man had to sell most of his possessions and was left with a chair without a back; a rickety table; one cot; no bedding; no fire for food; and his own nakedness. His wife and family was barely covered. The reporter stated: 'To see, on a bitterly cold winter evening, four children lying on the floor around their father's cot, and the poor mother, sitting on the only chair with an infant in her arms, fairly overcome for want of rest, trying to get a little sleep between her husband's paroxysms of coughing, was a sight not soon to be forgotten'.

The mission also ran a convalescent home for women at Weston-super-Mare.

In an *Occasional Paper*,[104] a visitor to the mission described a day's work at the dispensary. On Mondays, Wednesdays, and Fridays all the workers assembled in the doctor's room and began the day with prayer for a blessing on their work. Meanwhile, the doors opened at 10 a.m., the patients admitted by the housekeeper until 10.45 a.m., the hour for the service, when the doors were closed, and no more patients, as a rule, were admitted during the day, attendance at the service being *sine qua non*. The patients assembled in rows, according to the order in which they were to see the doctor. The service commenced at a quarter to eleven and lasted about twenty minutes. The harmonium was played, and a short gospel message was given by the doctor or some Christian friend. They then, in order, saw the doctor. After, they proceed to the dispensary with their prescriptions and bottles, which were dealt with by the lady dispensers. Meanwhile, the patients were entertained by the singing of Ira Sankey's hymns.

The perfect order and quiet maintained throughout were remarkable, as was the interest taken by each patient and the considerate way in which their wants were supplied. Clothes were often handed out, and every day, the doctor, ladies, and nurse were busily employed visiting patients at their homes. The secret appears to be much prayer.

The Medical Mission was still in existence in Redcross street until its work was taken over by the National Health Service.

Homoeopathic Dispensaries

A homoeopathic dispensary was opened in 1852 in Queen Square, and the first medical officer was Dr Macintosh. The next year the dispensary was removed to Upper Berkeley Place and then to the Triangle in Clifton.

In 1883 Miss Charles of Clifton contributed £1,000 through Dr Morgan and Miss Rich (also of Clifton), £100 through Dr Nicholson, towards the founding of a homoeopathic hospital. In the same year, 7 Brunswick Square, together with the adjoining Pembroke Cottage, the latter being used as a dispensary in addition to the dispensary which was already carried out at the Triangle. In 1884 Miss Charles gave a further sum of £1,000 for the furthering of homeopathic treatment. Additional information on the homoeopathic dispensaries can be found in *Homoeopathy in Bristol 1840–1925*.[105]

The Redland Dispensary

The Redland Dispensary was established in 1860 and was sited in 3 Grove Buildings, just off Whiteladies Road. It used the standard subscriber note system and then became part provident institution, whereby the subscriber note – one's own or one's patron's – bought a month's treatment.[106] The dispensary was funded by church collections, other contributions, and legacies.

In 1862 a newspaper advertisement indicated that Mr B Maurice had resigned as the RMO and a replacement was required – the note was signed by George M Stansfeld honorary secretary.[107] He was Bristol's first factory doctor. Benjamin Maurice was a surgeon, the son of a Westbury-on-Trym surgeon and grandson of an apothecary who practised at St Michael's Hill.

In 1863 Mr Webster advertised that he would see deaf patients at no charge on Fridays at 11 a.m. at the Redland Dispensary and his private patients at 2 p.m.

The dispensary was still working in 1900.[108] The notice says attendance for general patients was on Tuesdays and Thursdays at 3 p.m. For patients with diseases of the eye, ear, and throat, hours were on Fridays.

Institution for the Cure of Deafness and Diseases of the Ear

This was established at 1 Lower Berkeley Place in 1851, where the surgeon was Mr JS Metford. The days of attendance were Sundays from 9 to 10.30 a.m. and Thursdays 9.30 to 11 a.m. Advice to the poor was gratis, and this continued to 1862, by which 623 cases had been

91

treated.[109] By 1864, the advertisements about the Clifton Dispensary for the cure of deafness no longer mentioned 'gratuitous'.

Matthews Directory of 1900 advertised that the institution was now at 12 Lower Berkeley Place, the surgeon was Mr Clement David Hailes, MD, FRCS, and the day of attendance for new patients was Thursday 9.30 to 11 a.m.

Ear Institution

Another dispensary for ear diseases opened at 13 Orchard Street for the cure of deafness and diseases of the ear, gratis to the poor, on Fridays at 1 p.m., where the surgeon was Mr M Downing.

The Read Dispensary for Women and Children

Lucy Read, born in 1834 in Essex, was the youngest child of a silk broker. She never married and moved with her widowed mother to Bristol in the middle of the nineteenth century. She lived in West Mall, Clifton. In 1878 she wrote to *The Times*[110] about her new dispensary:

> It was the knowledge that many of the most respectable women of the poor allow ailments to become aggravated maladies before they will endure the publicity of the hospitals or run the risk of the young dispensary doctors that led me to introduce myself to Dr Eliza W Dunbar, who had settled here, and to ask her to give gratuitous advice to the poor. She consented … and has lately had no fewer than fifty-three patients in one morning. Women come from all parts of Bristol, from the neighbouring villages, and even from other towns.

Dunbar was previously excluded from the Children's Hospital in 1874 when she was known as Eliza Walker.

The dispensary started in 1874. In 1900,[111] it was open every day (except Sunday) from 11.30 a.m. to 12.30 p.m. and was supported by voluntary contributions and payment by patients. The honorary medical attendants were Eliza W Dunbar, MD; Emily Eberle, MA, FRCS; and Marion Linton, BA, MB. There were two male doctors giving support: honorary consulting physician Shingleton Smith, who subsequently became the first professor of medicine in Bristol, and the honorary surgeon W Harsant.

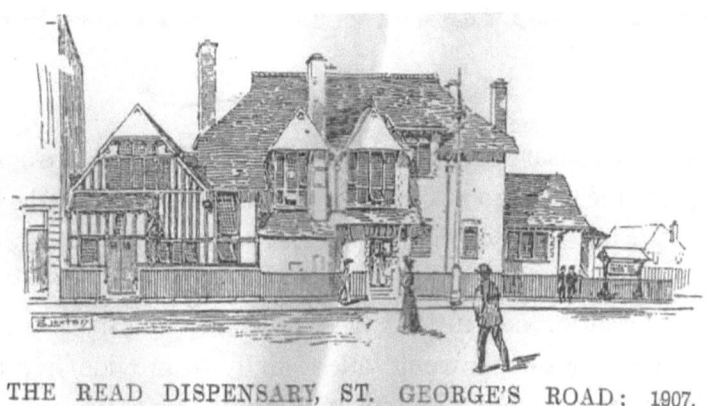

THE READ DISPENSARY, ST. GEORGE'S ROAD; 1907.

Image of the Read Dispensary courtesy
of Bristol Reference Library

Eliza Dunbar became registered as a doctor in 1877 – having previously been working with her Zurich medical qualification. Apparently, she had always wanted to open her own hospital, and in 1895, she was able to open the Bristol Private Hospital for Women and Children in Berkeley Square, Clifton. It was initially for twelve patients and met the needs of that class of woman for whom a large public hospital was obviously unsuitable – for instance, those engaged in teaching and business. It would have 'greater privacy and more refined surroundings'.[112] It subsequently moved to Clifton Down Road.

Chapter 5

THE LONDON DISPENSARIES

The first dispensary ever to be created in Britain resulted from a letter sent from the Common Council of the City of London to the College of Physicians in November 1696, drawing the college's attention to the pressing need for medical services for the sick poor.[113] A plan had been put forward in 1675 to provide a dispensary at the college where two physicians would attend daily to provide free medical advice to the sick poor. The Society of Apothecaries were approached to provide any medicines prescribed at inexpensive charges, but no agreement was reached. In 1687 the college declared that all members of the college would give free medical advice to poor people within the city and seven miles around. In 1696, the college decided by a narrow majority to provide a store of medicines that would be supplied at cost. Each physician on the committee agreed to contribute £10 to start the scheme. A dispensary was opened the next year in the college buildings in Warwick Lane and was very popular, with more than four thousand prescriptions being issued a year. Branch dispensaries were opened in St Martin's Lane and St Peter's Alley, Cornhill. There was no home visiting, and the opposing forces within the college forced the dispensaries to close in 1725.

The next dispensary was opened in 1769 by Dr George Armstrong. This was exclusively for the sick children of the poor and was initially in Red Lion Square, Holborn. In 1772 Armstrong wrote: 'This charity has now been three years on foot, during which time medicines and advice have been administered gratis and without letters of recommendation to about 3,300 children of necessitous parents'.

He personally bore most of the expense of running the dispensary in its early years, and in addition to prescribing for the sick children, Armstrong made it his business to educate the parents on diet, hygiene, and clothing. The charity closed in 1781.

The first of the successful, well-established, and well-staffed dispensaries was created as the General Dispensary, Aldersgate Street in 1770 with one hundred subscribers.

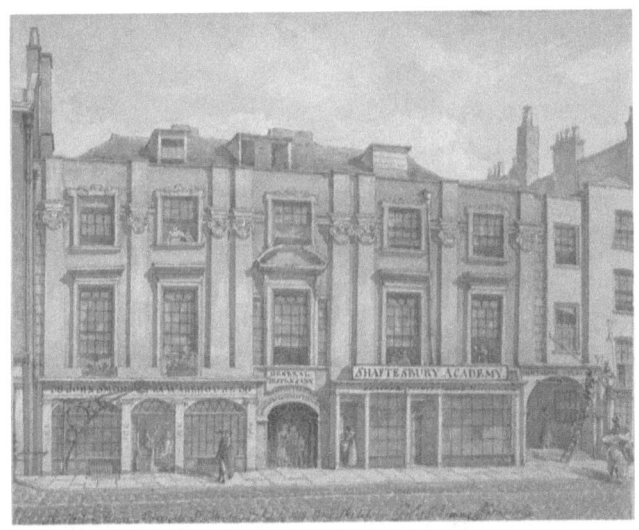

The General Dispensary, Aldersgate Street
View of Shaftesbury House, including Shaftesbury Academy, general dispensary, and John Smith's Tea Warehouse, with figures and a lamplighter, 1819. Watercolour by Robert Blemmell Schnebbelie (1792–1849). Image courtesy of Guildhall Library, City of London with permission.

One of its first physicians, Dr John Coakley Lettsom, wrote[114]

'I have attended nearly 1,700 poor persons, into many of whose habitations I have entered and been conversant with their sufferings. Sometimes, indeed, by successive attacks of illness, they are incapable of procuring the common necessaries of life; they have literally wanted bread, as well as clothes.'

He also remarked on the professional advantage of being a physician to a dispensary: 'By my election to the general dispensary, a more extensive field of practice afforded me daily opportunities of ascertaining the doubts and clearing up the difficulties under which I had laboured'.

The Quaker doctor Lettsom trained as a physician, surgeon, and apothecary and, besides his philanthropy, is remembered for his extensive garden in South London, his knowledge of botany, and as the founder of the interdisciplinary Medical Society of London in 1773. One of his case studies is memorable. It took place in 1780 and was a visit he made in Little Greenwich. He wrote:

> 'With difficulty, I found my way up a dark passage to a little chamber, furnished with one bedstead and a worn-out blanket, which constituted the only couch whereon this afflicted family could recline their heads to rest; and what a scene did they present! Near the centre of the bed lay the mother, incapable of telling her complaints. The spittle had dried upon her lips, which, as well as her gums were covered with a black crust – the concomitant symptoms of a putrid fever, the disorder under which she laboured, in its most malign state'.

Two children about twelve and five years old, both with a high fever, shared the same bed, along with another two-year-old, all almost naked, and crying out for water. A four-year-old was the only family member capable of fetching it. The mother and one of the children had large, untreated bed sores. Lettsom's timely intervention saved the family. He arranged for proper medical care, paid a neighbour to come in and nurse the household, and secured financial help from the parish churchwardens.

The medical staff of the general dispensary consisted of three physicians and three surgeons; one physician and one surgeon attended the dispensary each day from one to four hours while the others visited the poor residing in any part of the city, whenever the severity of the disease precluded the patient's personal attendance at the institution.

The licensed apothecary resided at the dispensary and was not allowed to engage in private practice, although he could take apprentices to learn the trade and assist him. He was required to dispense all medicines and attend emergencies during the day or night until a surgeon or physician arrived. His duties were so arduous that he was later provided with an assistant, who received £30, and a porter receiving £38 per annum. Hodgkinson[115] adds that the complete separation of duties, between the prescribers of medicines and the dispenser, was of utmost importance to the poor, because the temptation to supply remedies that were at hand and the easiest to prepare was removed, and the best drugs could be ordered without regard for the trouble that might be required in their preparation. No restriction was placed on the liberal use of expensive medicines, and it was maintained that they were as good as any administered to the wealthy.

In 1844 each patient cost 1s and 11½ pence on average. This calculation was derived from the following information given to the select committee on Poor Law Medical Relief, 1844:

Table 12   Details of Expenditure and Workload of Aldersgate Street Dispensary in 1844

Expenditure			Cost (£-s-d)	Cost (£-s-d)
Drugs, wine, chemicals etc			360-13-8	
Salaries	Apothecary	£120.00		
	Assistant	£30.00		

	Poundage to Collector	£18-6-6		
	Porter	£62-8-0	230-14-6	
Incidentals	Furniture, advertising, stationery, fuel, rent etc	£189-16-10	189-16-10	£781-5-0
Total Expenses				£814-2-6
Amount of Relief Given				
Attendances at Dispensary	By Physicians	17976		
	By Surgeons	6325	24301	
Visits at homes of poor			4662	
Visits at doctors' houses			8295	
Repeat medicines, not seen by doctor			6000	
Total				43256
Average number receiving medicine per day		138		
Number of times each person seen by doctor		4.5		
Number of times receives medicine		5.22		
Therefore, average cost of materials to individual		10¼d		
Labour in preparing and dispensing them		6¼d		
Rent, firing, to each individual		7d		
Total		1s 11½d		

This Aldersgate Street Dispensary survived until 1932 when it was absorbed by St Bartholomew's Hospital.[116]

Other dispensaries quickly sprang up in London:

Westminster General (Soho)   1774
The London Dispensary (Artillery St) 1777
Surrey Dispensary (Union St)   1777
Metropolitan Dispensary (Fore St)   1779

Finsbury Dispensary	1780
Eastern Dispensary Whitechapel	1782
St Marylebone General	1785
Public Dispensary (Carey St)	1783
Western Dispensary (Westminster)	1789
City Dispensary (Grocers Hall Court)	1792

By 1802, dispensaries in London were serving fifty thousand poor patients annually over an area of fifty square miles round the city. Most of the dispensaries made special provision for smallpox inoculation and later, vaccination.[117]

The Westminster Dispensary

The early minutes of this dispensary indicate that nineteen men met at the Adelphi Tavern on 6 June 1774 and proposed that a dispensary be set up in Westminster where 'eminent and experienced physicians will be appointed to attend the patients in their own homes. A house will be taken for a dispensary where the apothecary who is to dispense the medicines directed by the physicians and to receive letters of recommendation from the Governors, shall constantly reside. A physician will attend at the dispensary every day from one o'clock to three, to give advice to such patients as are able to go there'.[118]

The Turk's Head Tavern at 9 Gerrard Street was purchased and the Westminster Dispensary founded.

In 1783 a salary of £50 a year was agreed to be paid to each physician, man-midwife, and surgeon; this salary was raised to £100 per annum in 1786.

In 1777 Dr John Millar published his *Observations on the Practice in the Medical Department of the Westminster General Dispensary*[119]. He describes the first two years' work at the dispensary where they saw 2,553 patients, among whom 515 suffered from consumption, 404 from remitting fever, 224 from stomach complaints, 189 from rheumatism, and 112 from venereal disease. The dispensary recruited midwives to deliver women in their own homes. The rate of pay was two shillings for each delivery.

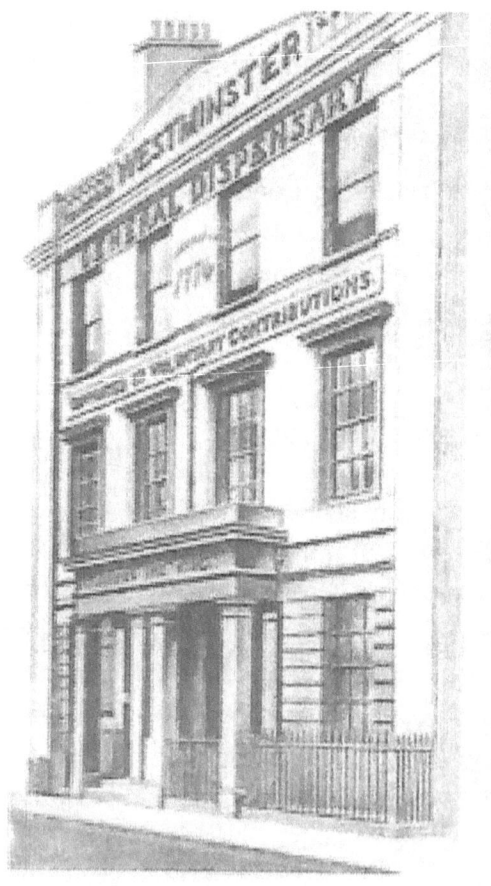

The Westminster Dispensary. Illustration from
The Chemist and Druggist 29 June 1957.

The apothecary dispensed medicines from 8 a.m. to 9 a.m.; from noon to 3 p.m., and from 6 to 7 p.m., and the costs of medicines were always carefully monitored. In 1903, for instance, 7,288 patients were treated at an average cost per patient of seven pence, and in 1908, the cost was reduced to five pence per patient with 9,759 treated.

Concern about the financial viability of the dispensary occurred in 1894[120] when subscriptions fell from £195 to £186 and there was a need for extensive property repairs. The treasurer was forced to loan the dispensary £100 of his own money to tide it over the difficulty. In the first decade of the twentieth century, the dispensary was amalgamated with the St George's and St James's Dispensary.

The Surrey Dispensary

The dispensary was situated in Union Street, Southwark, and the 1822 book of *Rules, Orders, and Regulations* indicates that it was an extremely well organised dispensary.[121] Its income each year exceeded £1,600, and it had a balance of more than £4000, with a rent to pay on premises of less than £50. It had three physicians, two surgeons, and one resident apothecary. The dispensary was created in 1777, and in 1822 had no fewer than seven members of Parliament as vice presidents! It was created to 'attend lying-in women and administer advice and medicines to the poor inhabitants of the borough of Southwark and places adjacent at the dispensary and at their own habitations'. It had three main committees: a committee of twenty-one governors who met monthly and to which doctors were only invited when required. There was a medical committee of fourteen physicians and surgeons who had to inspect the drugs and give advice to the monthly and audit committees, and an audit committee of nine members who had to examine all bills before payment.

One of the physicians attended the dispensary every day (except Sundays) at 11 a.m. to 'write for the outpatients', and then they visited the home patients. Their pupils could also attend but could not prescribe. There was a printed pharmacopoeia. There was also a paid secretary and collector.

Each year there was an anniversary dinner to help publicise the institution and to raise funds. The price of tickets was twelve shillings, which included the cost of the dinner, and should not exceed 9s 6d (this had to include dessert and porter). The cost of the professional singers was not to exceed £10. The clergy who had preached sermons about the dispensary in order to raise funds, the medical gentlemen and the apothecary and his assistant, and the collector were all guests at the dinner. During the year, 4,195 patients were seen and 3,243 were cured. Of these, 1,398 had been visited in their homes.

The Surrey Dispensary paid gratuities to its physicians and surgeons amounting to £262 10s during the year. The apothecary was paid £149 2s, including cost of coals and candles, and his assistant received a salary of £35. The cost of medicines was £342 16s, and the midwives received £115 10s.

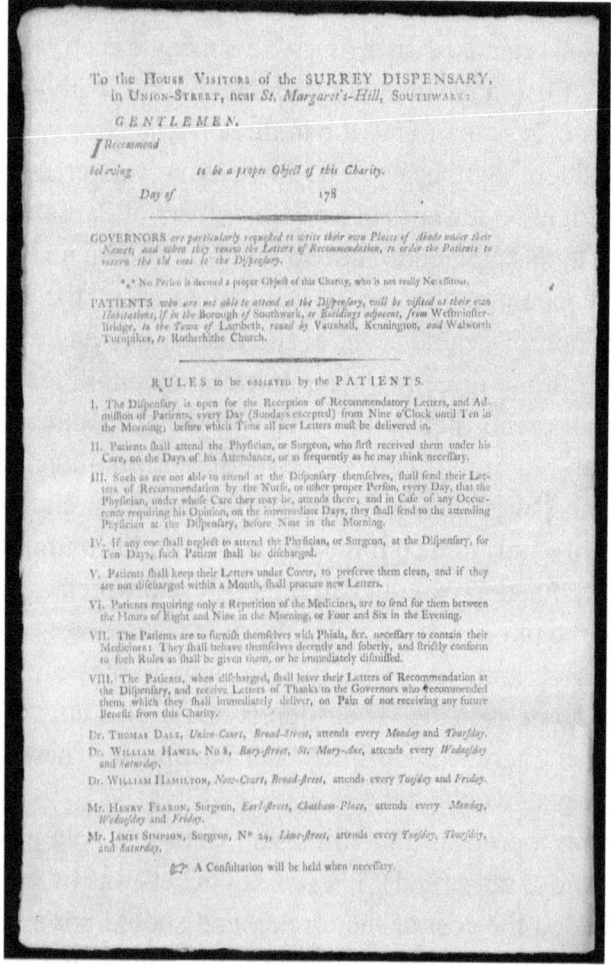

One of the letters of recommendation to the Surrey
Dispensary courtesy Wellcome Library.

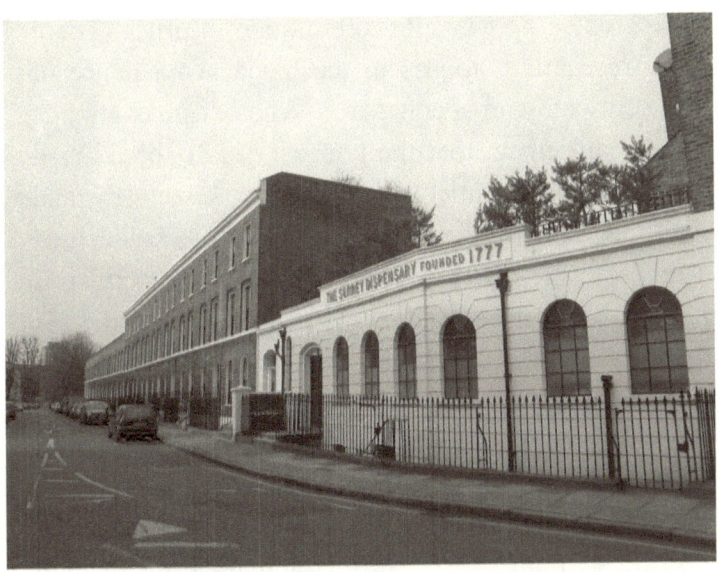

'The Surrey Dispensary now a private
residence courtesy Ben Jones

Towards the end of the nineteenth century the relationship between
the committee and the doctors in the Surrey Dispensary appears to
have deteriorated. In 1894, *The Lancet* included an editorial about
the dispensary.[122]

'The committee of management of the Surrey
Dispensary … have recently revised the rules of
the institution. We would call attention to the new
and revised regulations affecting the medical and
surgical staff, upon whom, of course, the utility of the
dispensary depends. Some of these regulations strike
us as unnecessary, others as positively inequitable
and oppressive. The change in tenure of office to a
maximum of ten years and subject to an annual re-
election might under exceptional circumstances be
useful, but it can hardly be questioned that under this
arrangement the dispensary might lose the services
of a medical officer just at a time when his age and

experience best fit him to continue in office. There are restrictions too as to the place of residence of the two surgeon-accoucheurs. Another innovation is the requirement that the honorary staff should visit patients at the patients' homes when necessary, and although the resident medical officer may be deputed to perform this duty the physicians and surgeons will be held responsible for the cases so treated. This increase in their duties and responsibilities is hardly likely to be accepted by the honorary staff without a protest, and we very much doubt if many in the future will care to undertake an office that demands so much expenditure of time and labour. It is almost adding insult to injury to provide that these officers shall each be granted fifty guineas annually "in order to meet any expenses that may be incurred in the course of their visiting duties or otherwise", and not only so, but the sum shall only be granted by the committee "after fully considering the nature and manner of performance of their duties". We opine that few, if any, professional gentlemen will consent to have their work criticised and appraised by a body of laymen, who in this manner would degrade their calling to the level of a trade, and estimate the remuneration in question on the principle of quid pro quo. We sincerely trust, for the credit of this old-established charity at least, that this obnoxious provision will be struck out before the new rules are finally adopted'.

This editorial provoked a letter from John Ince, MD, a retired Indian army surgeon who had been a resident surgeon at the dispensary from 1854–6.[123] He was a member of the subcommittee that drafted the revised rules that *The Lancet* had commented on. He wrote:

'Some of the members of staff have been attached to the dispensary from twenty to forty years. As to the outpatients, many complaints as to irregularity of attendance have from time to time been received by the committee of management, and the attendance book of the staff fully sustained them. Patients have been kept waiting as much as from two the three hours, and when the medical officers have arrived the patients have been rapidly disposed of at the rate of from fifty to seventy an hour; sometimes five or six being in the consulting room at the same time, and in one case a female patient complained of being obliged to expose her chest for examination in the presence of others. As to the home patients, those unable to attend as outpatients, the subscribers, are led by the rules to expect that these patients shall be visited by the physicians and surgeons, and in former years this was so, but of late this duty has been transferred to the resident medical officer. An official return before me shows that for the years 1892 and 1893, they only attended about 10 per cent of them. As to the lying-in department of the charity, the rules require that "all difficult labours should be attended by the surgeon accoucheurs". During 1892 and 1893, they only attended 10 per cent – the remaining 90 per cent being left to the resident medical officers. The truth is that under the old rules, the committee have no due authority over the staff, a state of things that cannot surely be defended. The new rules are intended as a rod, not necessarily for frequent use, but as a symbol always'.

Dr Hooper, the senior physician at the dispensary, replied to Dr Ince's comments and in two letters claimed that Dr Ince was out of touch with the work of the dispensary. He explained that the work of the dispensary extended over a very large area, and it was impractical for the honorary physicians and surgeons to visit over that area. He contrasted the visiting area with the Finsbury Dispensary that had a much more restricted visiting area. Dr Hooper stated that he had not the smallest objection to the governors having authority over the staff, but he wrote, 'I think we have a right to be treated and written to as innocent men until we are found to be guilty'.[124]

The Royal Kent Dispensary

This was founded in 1783, and the Miller Hospital was added to the rear of the dispensary in 1881.[125] The original dispensary was situated in the Broadway, Deptford, and in 1787, the rules stated that there should be six visiting districts:

1. the two parishes of Deptford
2. Greenwich
3. Woolwich and Charlton
4. Lewisham and Lee
5. from Rotherhive church to Deptford
6. from Camberwell church to Deptford

The physician attended at the dispensary on Tuesdays and Fridays, supervised the direction for the outpatients, and visited house patients when requested by any of the medical assistants. His pupils had the liberty to attend with him but were not allowed to perform chirurgical operations. The surgeons and medical assistants visited patients when they couldn't get to the dispensary, assisted in difficult labours, and attended such women after delivery. The two Deptford surgeons were house surgeons at the dispensary and attended there alternatively every morning from nine to ten o'clock or longer if necessary, to examine and order medicine for all who came under their care. For any capital operation they had to get the approval of the physician, and in difficult surgical cases all the surgeons were consulted.

In 1796 Thomas Forbes Leith, MD FRS, was the physician, and there were nine visiting surgeons. Mr GM Jones was the resident apothecary. By 1836, the medical establishment had increased to a physician and thirteen surgeons and medical assistants, 'all of whom served the charity gratuitously and from motives of humanity'. In a report in 1830[126], it was stated that no medical lectures were ever given in the dispensary as 'it was not conducive to give lectures such as those that were given in the Surrey Dispensary and other kindred institutions'. It was further stated that such lectures were an important means of medical education about that time.

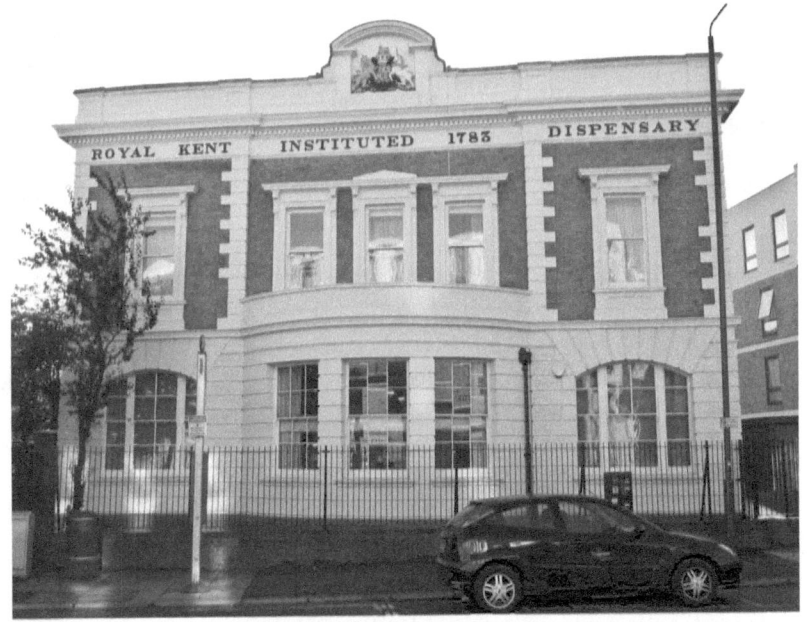

The Royal Kent Dispensary
courtesy Nige B

Loudon[127] compared the level of staffing of several dispensaries, including the Royal Kent Dispensary, Whitehaven, Exeter, Newcastle-upon-Tyne and the Bristol Dispensary and demonstrated the considerable variation in the staff numbers of the dispensaries see Table 13.

Table 13   Staffing levels in selected dispensaries (after Loudon)

Dispensary	Bristol Dispensary	Royal Kent	Exeter	Whitehaven	Newcastle-upon-Tyne
Year in which data applied	1805	1815	1827	1802	1790
Physicians	3	1	6	1	7
Surgeons	0	10	6	1	1
Apothecaries	2	1*	1 (dispenser)	1	1
Accoucheurs	3				
Consulting physician and surgeons			3	1	
Total admissions	About 1000	About 2500	1049	6100**	1964
Home visits	NK	About 350	NK	595	NK
Annual income of dispensary	£3-400 (in 1791)	£1,200.00	£504 (in 1839)	£321.00	£4,900.00

NK = no record

* assistant apothecary also employed

**In 1791 there were 3,721 admissions. According to M Sydney[128], there were 2,057 admissions in 1783.

Financial problems in 1831 resulted in the two house surgeons' duties being taken over gratuitously by local surgeons, but they were paid fees if called urgently to midwifery cases.

The year 1837 was momentous for the charity as the Duke of Wellington chaired the annual meeting, and the newly crowned Queen Victoria became the patron of the dispensary. It was said that if a larger room could have been obtained there would have been more than three times the number of subscribers present to hear the great man.

In 1841 a very serious difference of opinion sprang up between the members of the medical committee and the monthly committee that led to the resignation of sixteen members of the medical staff.

However, things quickly returned to normal. Mr Henley, the apothecary, resigned in 1843 after forty-three years of faithful service and was granted an annuity of £50. In 1851, new premises had to be found, and the dispensary moved from the Broadway, Deptford, location to Greenwich Road, and the new dispensary cost £2,954. In 1856, the twenty surgeons of the dispensary circulated a letter to all neighbouring doctors inviting them to form a medical society based in the dispensary where there would be monthly educational meetings. Further developments included the establishing the Miller Memorial Hospital behind the dispensary, and in 1890 a branch dispensary was opened at 313 High Road, Lee.

Canon John Miller, after whom the hospital was named, was the originator of the Hospital Sunday mass contributions whilst he was the vicar of a Birmingham church. For the second half of his ministry he became vicar of Greenwich and made a big impression on the local population. Hospital Sunday occurred each year, and churches were encouraged to take up a collection for dispensaries and hospitals. In London, this was collected and distributed by a committee,[129] and some members of the dispensary committee felt they obtained an inappropriately small proportion of the fund each year as their local churches stopped their regular collections for their local dispensary, assuming the annual Hospital Sunday collection was all that was necessary.

The Finsbury Dispensary

This was opened in a 'large and handsome house' on St John's Street, Clerkenwell in 1780.[130] In 1828 it was reported that nearly 150,000 persons had been helped by the institution and that about 4000 people were seen for the first time each year. The average number of people under care at any one time was 600. The report stated that 'although hospitals are excellent establishments, they are difficult to access, patients are admitted only on one day of the week, fees are required, the patients is taken from the bosom of his family and the nurses are strangers. The blessings to the poor themselves are many and important. Application for medical aid, on the first feelings of indisposition, prevents the spreading of many contagious disorders, and pestilence … is strangled in its birth'.

According to the rules and regulations of the dispensary in 1841, each governor was entitled to fifteen letters of recommendation per one guinea subscribed and that the committee of thirty governors was chosen annually from the subscribers. The patron was King Leopold I of Belgium, and there were two physicians and one surgeon; one of the physicians attended the dispensary two mornings each week and the surgeon three. The dispensary was open daily (except Sundays) from noon until two and from four until six o'clock. The apothecary resided in the house for the purpose of compounding and dispensing for the patients and attended to the patients in the absence of the medical officers in emergencies. He was not allowed to have private patients.

By the early twentieth century, the notes for the Finsbury Dispensary, which had moved from the original site, had become quite detailed.

FINSBURY DISPENSARY,

FRIEND STREET, GOSWELL ROAD, E.C.1.

LETTER OF RECOMMENDATION.

I recommend
Patient's Name..

„   Address..

as a proper person to receive Medical Attendance or Foot Treatment
from this Institution.

Governor's Name..

Residence..

Date............................*19...*

MEDICAL OFFICERS:
Honorary Consulting Physician:
Sir ERNEST GRAHAM-LITTLE, M.D., F.R.C.P., M.P.,
40, Wimpole Street, W.1.

Honorary Consulting Surgeon:
ARTHUR EVANS, Esq., O.B.E., M.S., M.D., F.R.C.S.,
86, Brook Street, W.1.

Resident Medical Officer:
AGNES B. SUTHERLAND, M.B., Ch.B.

Assistant Resident Medical Officer:
PATRICIA S. WARREN, M.B., Ch.B.

Monday and Friday at 9.30 a.m. and 6 p.m.
Tuesday, Wednesday and Thursday at 3 p.m.
Saturday at 12 NOON.

DIRECTIONS TO PATIENTS.

1.—The Dispensary is open :—

MONDAY,   9.30 a.m. to 12.30 p.m. and 6 p.m. to 8 p.m.
TUESDAY,   1 p.m. to 6 p.m.
WEDNESDAY, 1 p.m. to 6 p.m.
THURSDAY, 1 p.m. to 6 p.m.
FRIDAY,   9.30 a.m. to 12.30 p.m. and 6 p.m. to 8 p.m.
SATURDAY, 10 a.m. to 1.30 p.m.

2.—Patients desiring to be visited at home must send their letters to the Dispensary **before 9.30 a.m.**

3.—Patients visited at home must send for their medicine when the Dispensary is open.

4.—Each patient must provide bottles, &c., and obtain from the Porter either a sixpenny ticket for a week's medicine, or a threepenny ticket for a half-week's medicine, according to the quantity of medicine prescribed. When patients are visited at their own homes, they are required to pay one shilling per week for medicine.

FOOT TREATMENT.
Chiropody and Massage.
Miss M. K. BOYD, C.S.M.M.G., M.I.S.Ch.
Monday and Friday, 5 p.m. to 8 p.m.
Thursday, 3 p.m. to 6 p.m.

Letters of Recommendation are available for Two Months from date of issue.

ARTHUR W. PRIOR, *Secretary.*

Photo courtesy London Metropolitan Archives (Acc/3778/001).

When patients were discharged they were required to give a letter of thanks to the Governor, or they would not receive any further help.

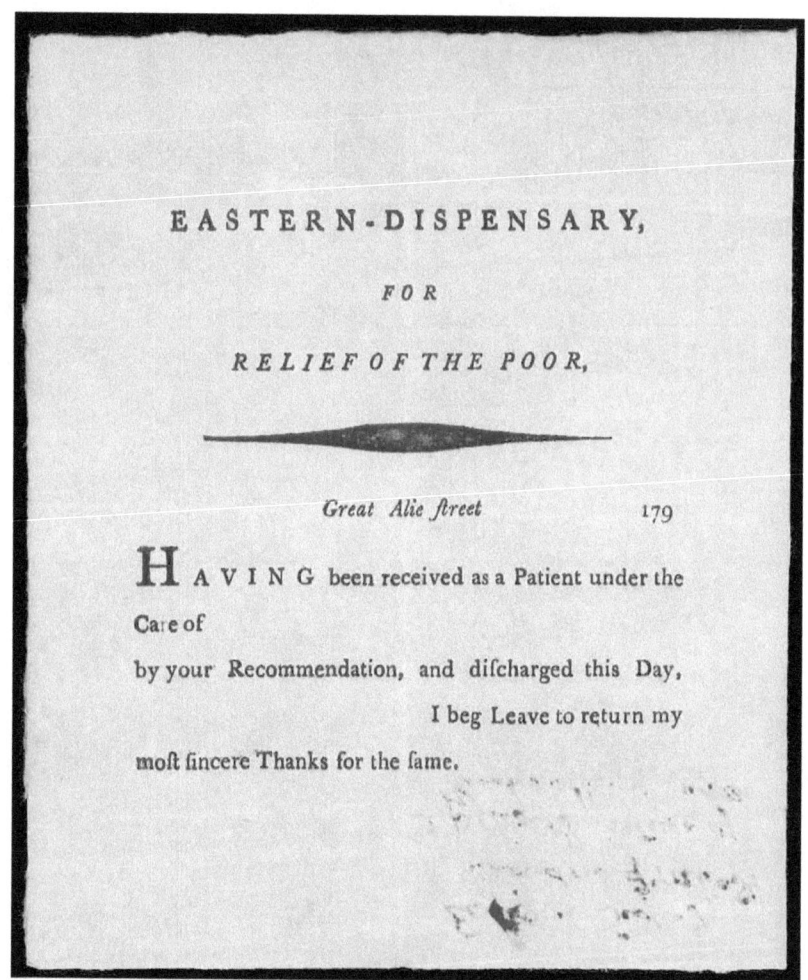

EASTERN-DISPENSARY,

FOR

RELIEF OF THE POOR,

Great Alie ſtreet   179

HAVING been received as a Patient under the Care of

by your Recommendation, and diſcharged this Day,

I beg Leave to return my moſt ſincere Thanks for the ſame.

A letter of thanks that patients were encouraged to give to the Subscriber who had recommended them to the dispensary (in this case at the Eastern dispensary). Photo courtesy Wellcome Library.

The Carey Street Dispensary

The Minute Book of the Public Dispensary on Carey Street, situated in Lincoln's Inn between the cities of London and Westminster,[131] states that the doctors received considerably more financial reward for their responsibilities than in most other dispensaries. On the first page of the Minutes in May 1796, it was recommended that the physician, Dr Willan, be given a gratuity of 50 guineas 'for his great attention to the patients, and the furtherance of the institution'. It was customary to give a similar donation to the surgeon, and these gratuities were repeated annually. The apothecary was paid £80 a year from 1804 with an annual allowance of £20 for coals and candles.

Life for the apothecary was not easy, and in January 1802 a committee investigated the fact that on some occasions he had addressed the patients with harshness and incivility. In one case he had omitted a material part of the physician's prescription and had neglected to give directions how to take a medicine after the prescription was changed.

Another entry in the Minutes was a letter from Mrs Elizabeth Haig:

> 'I'd had the favour of being in this dispensary for some time [as] a patient of Surgeon Pearson's, by whom I have found the greatest relief – not only in my health but also two of my wounds of my foot are healed. But I have suffered much violent pain lately not having a sufficient quantity of opium, it being rather a dear article, and my husband's stipend being so very small'.

After investigation, it was found that Mrs Haig was using large quantities of opium; her request was denied, and she was excluded from the dispensary.

In 1793[132] the medical staff was Robert Willan (physician), John Pearson (surgeon), and John Nelson (the resident apothecary). The physician attended the dispensary on Monday, Wednesday, and Friday at noon, and afterwards visited those patients unable to attend the dispensary. The surgeon attended on Tuesday and Thursday at eleven o'clock and visited afterwards. The apothecary attended to the house and compounded the medicines prescribed by the physician and surgeon and had no other employment. The dispensary also employed a collector and a secretary. The patients were required to attend at the specified times, to behave soberly, to conform to the rules, and to thank the subscriber after being discharged from the dispensary.

Robert Willan, who like Lettsom was a Quaker, remained physician for twenty-one years and had many eminent pupils working with him, including Richard Bright, who subsequently became a physician at the dispensary. Willan developed an interest in public health and, most famously, as it relates to skin disease. He wrote monthly reports that were published in the *Monthly Magazine*, which provided an account of the state of the weather and of the diseases most prevalent in London from 1796 to 1800. He drew attention to the fact that one common skin disease (psoriasis or *lepra vulgaris*) was due to exposure to cold and moisture and recommended that if there were better access to public bathhouses, many skin diseases would be prevented or relieved.[133]

The Bloomsbury Dispensary

During the first fifty years of the nineteenth century, London doubled its population from about 675,000, and the area around Great Russell Street and Bloomsbury became grossly overcrowded and full of poor-quality housing with the added complication of the building of a railway network in the area. The Bloomsbury Dispensary was created in 1801 to serve impoverished tradesmen, workmen, and servants, but not for the idle and improvident, and certainly not for those who could pay for medical aid.[134] In the records of that dispensary for 1868, the artisan workers who came for treatment included stonemasons, horsehair workers, cabinetmakers and joiners, gas fitters, and French polishers. Bronchial consumption and metallic poisoning were the result of inhalations from work of this sort and inevitably proved fatal.[135] The largest occupation for women was domestic service (nine out of ten employed as such).

At the end of the first ten years of the work of the Bloomsbury Dispensary 10,014 persons had been treated at the dispensary, of which 1,541 had been visited in their own homes. The dispensary was managed by committees: a medical committee, and another for canvassing new residents and for reminding the established residents that the dispensary needed their help. Another committee arranged for the preaching of charity sermons, and house visitors dealt with the premises. One of the other functions of the dispensary was to promote the cowpox vaccination to prevent smallpox, and Dr Edward Jenner used the Bloomsbury Dispensary for this purpose – he was designated superintendent of vaccine inoculation and remained on the medical committee until his death in 1823.

Details of case histories of patients were not recorded until 1846, and in 1867 the resident medical officer recorded the following table of diseases.

Table 14   Diseases treated at the Bloomsbury Dispensary in 1867

This table shows the large numbers of patients with respiratory and diarrhoeal complaints that were dealt with by the dispensary doctors:

Disease	No of cases	No of deaths
Smallpox	10	none
Scarlatina	14	3
Whooping Cough	35	1
Measles	45	3
Continued Fever	12	
Typhus	4	3
Typhoid	19	
Diseases of brain and Nervous system	41	5
Rheumatism and gout	186	
Heart diseases	70	2
Catarrh, bronchitis, and bronchopneumonia	488	23
Phthisis (pulmonary tuberculosis)	152	31
Haemoptysis (coughing blood)	17	

Diarrhoea (simple)	6	
Cholera and choleraic diarrhoea	892	2
Diseases of liver	43	
Diseases of kidney	23	2
Atrophy	11	9
Cancer	13	3
Croup, rickets, caries of spine and natural decay	4	4

A new, purpose-built dispensary was opened in 1881. In 1921 contributions were asked from patients for the first time, and a sixpence fee provided a week's supply of medicine, but insured patients were asked to pay one shilling per visit. In 1940 the premises were hit by a high-explosive bomb, and another bomb destroyed the remains of the building the next year.

The Western General Dispensary

Following the rapid increase in the population of the area to the west of Baker Street in 1830 that was associated with the building of the Great Western Railway, poverty and overcrowding became a major problem, and this institution was planned for the sick poor of St Marylebone, Paddington, and Kilburn.[136] The men involved in starting this dispensary included a relatively large number of doctors, four general practitioners, and a physician, with eight laymen and the curate of the parish Revd Bryant Burgess, who took the chair at the original meeting. A house was purchased at 9 Lisson Grove South, and the objects of the charity were

- to provide medical and surgical advice and medicine for poor persons, without residential limitations;
- to provide attendance by medical officers for patients in their homes if they reside within one mile of the institution;
- to provide beds in the dispensary house for sufferers from accidents in the immediate neighbourhood; and

- to supply wine, sago, and arrowroot for those patients whose poverty and ill health require it.

The medical staff consisted of two consulting surgeons and two consulting physicians with four honorary medical officers for the regular work. Two of these medical officers attended the dispensary every day except Sunday, and they visited patients in their homes. Schuster commented that 'The governors considered it a great advantage to have general practitioners, with their intimate knowledge of the locality, doing this voluntary work. They were keen, well-qualified men, filled with zeal for curing their impecunious patients'.[137]

The medical officers acted primarily as surgeons until 1841, when it was decided to have two physicians and three surgeons, an arrangement which proved a great success. By degrees, the general practitioner principle lapsed, and in 1882 the honorary staff were all FRCS or MRCP (that is, qualified as specialists). There was also a dispenser/secretary (paid £50 per year) who was resident in the house. He was always on call to see patients when they arrived, kept notes and compounded and dispensed medicines. In 1840 this apothecary was relieved of his secretarial duties and allowed to have an apprentice, who could attend the local medical school and gain a medical qualification. Other paid staff included a housekeeper (paid £15 per year) who cooked for the dispenser, a porter and a collector, who was allowed to keep 5 per cent of the contributions he obtained. A collector who resigned in 1920 after fifty years' service was then made a director.

The Western General did not escape dissension between the committee and the doctors. In the early 1830s one of the medical officers, Mr Flood, was criticised for sending a substitute to do his work without permission from the committee. He wrote an indignant reply, and the committee withdrew their complaint, but Flood resigned. Surprisingly, he was appointed co-treasurer with Revd Burgess and began making serious charges against the treasurer. He wrote at the end of a letter to the committee where he asked for all committee members to resign: 'I cannot but lament that the cause of the charity is committed to the care of men who … can betray a degree of stupidity and ignorance not to be equalled in any civilized country'.

Flood disappeared from the scene in 1834.

The dispensary had its own pharmacopoeia and it was examined by the Committee from time to time with a view to cutting down costs. The medicines included aperients, expectorants, liniments, quinine, iron, and cod liver oil. This last item was prescribed in great quantity as it had, in the 1840s, become a favourite remedy for rickets and consumption, and £52 was spent on it in 1850. Dr CJB Williams (consulting physician to the dispensary) wrote in 1849 that cod liver oil was a 'more beneficial treatment for pulmonary consumption than any agent, medicinal, dietetic, or regimental, that has yet been employed'. Even earlier, two other consulting physicians at the dispensary had made a trial of cod liver oil treatment, so it was not surprising that it was a popular remedy.

The dispensary decided to provide six accident beds in 1835, three for males on the first floor and three for women on the second, where there was also a small operating room. Medical cases were admitted after 1841, and in 1843 a midwifery service for the district was started. Between 1845 and 1854 the average cost per patient was calculated to be 3s 6d in 1845 but had fallen to just under one shilling in 1854, due to the fact that in that year the inpatient part of the dispensary closed, apart for two beds that were kept for emergencies. This followed discussions between the dispensary directors and the directors of the new St Mary's Hospital, which opened in 1851 when a merger between the two institutions was considered. This did not take place, as the important function of home visiting would have been lost. Twenty years later, in 1873, the new building was erected close by in Cosway Street.

After 1880, new departments started opening in the dispensary: ophthalmology in 1883; ENT in 1891; and a children's department in 1920. A radiographer was appointed in 1908 and a chiropodist in 1924.

The committee often debated whether the dispensary should become a provident institution, but on three separate occasions (1839, 1869, and 1873) the idea was rejected. The directors considered that the public were genuinely too poor to make provident contributions and belonged to a class that lay between the 'stable artisan' and the 'depraved pauper'. They had not even consented to a suggestion sent by the British Medical Association in 1894 that they should adopt a means test, believing, as they did, that the service was not abused.[138]

In 1936 the St Marylebone General Dispensary started negotiating for a union with the dispensary, as they were looking for a new building, and, in effect, the St Marylebone Dispensary took over the work of the Western General.

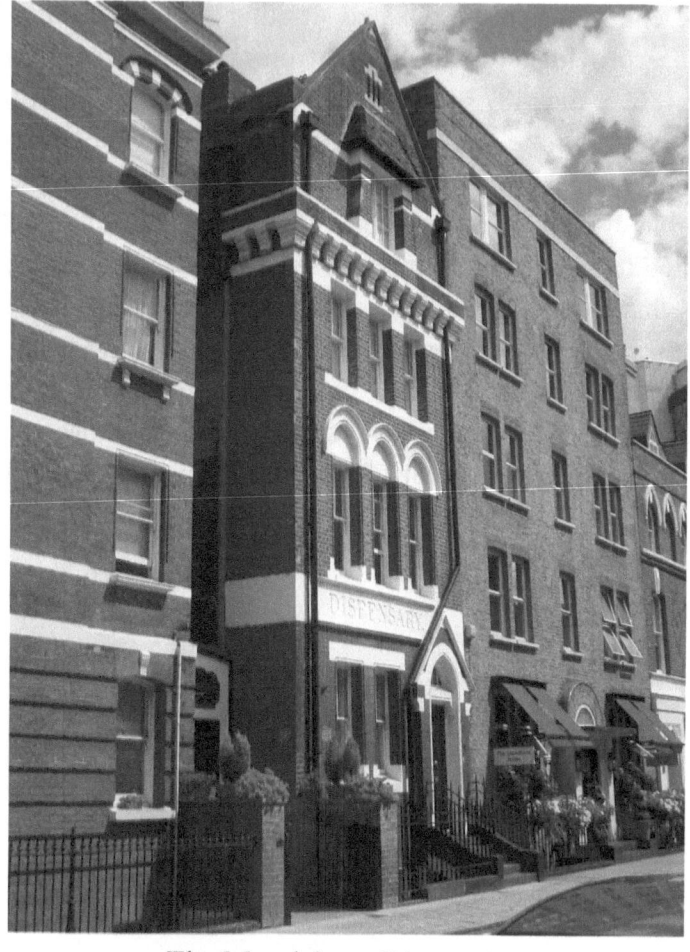

The Marylebone Dispensary
courtesy of Jamie Barras

The Western General Dispensary shared the characteristics of the two large Bristol Dispensaries in the loyalty of some families to care within the dispensary. Dr Edgar Barker, a doctor founder, with his son made up an overlapping sequence of association for 73 years as medical officers, treasurers and directors (1830-1893), (1857-1903) and Mr RJP Broughton, together with his son (HPB) served 93 years as directors and Chairmen of the Board (1853-1911, (1886-1946).

The Poor Law Dispensaries

The Metropolitan Poor Act 1867 provided for the establishment of dispensaries throughout London. The dispensaries were a great advance on the previously existing arrangements for the supply of outdoor medical relief. Instead of the medical officer having to supply medicines out of his own salary, they were now provided by the guardians and dispensed by a dispenser, giving his whole time to the work. The dispensaries were conveniently sited. The poor who were able to go to the dispensary were now certain of seeing the medical officer at a fixed hour every day. The system provided a better check on the medical officer's treatment of cases and secured a more effective control over the whole administration of outdoor relief. Contrary to expectation, the cost of providing a dispensary was found to be 'extremely small' – in many cases the dispensary was simply an ordinary dwelling house with a waiting room for patients built on the ground behind; or it was sometimes incorporated into other buildings such as an Infirmary. Poor Law dispensaries were later opened in several large urban centres away from London.[139]

The supporters of dispensaries in the second half of the eighteenth century were in direct competition with the hospitals. Lawrence[140] stated:

> Providing medical advice and inexpensive medicines to outpatients, with some home visits, had many advantages over inpatient care. Dispensaries assisted with the same sorts of illnesses, kept families together, fostered independence from excessive charity, prevented the spread of disease, and above all, were cheaper. They could help more patients per pound than hospitals. Donors and subscribers sprang up throughout the metropolis, and most of the hospitals already had, or then established, outpatient services to compete. The process continued into the nineteenth century.

Figure 1. Charitable and Provident Dispensary Provision in London 1770–1900.[141]

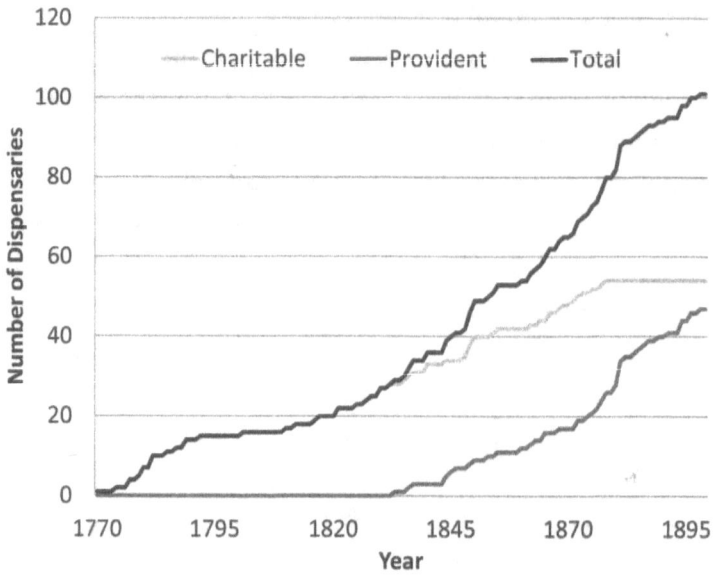

Chapter 6

DISPENSARIES IN ENGLAND AND WALES

Many dispensaries were created in England and Wales during the two centuries before the National Health Service was formed. Most lasted for many decades, some developed into hospitals, and all had their special features, which was not surprising as there was little communication between them, and they were all managed by local people.

The surgeon HW Rumsey, in his evidence to the select committee on the Poor Law Medical Service in 1844, criticized the irregular and uncertain attendance on dispensary patients at their own homes. In a few towns, patients were visited regularly by honorary physicians and surgeons, but, he said, it was not to be expected that any regular or extensive system of domiciliary visiting would be maintained by unpaid officers. In the majority of cases the paid resident apothecary was the sole visitor, and the honoraries only attended serious cases in the homes when specially requested to do so by the apothecary. Rumsey didn't believe that dispensary patients were as conscientiously treated as patients of the union medical officer. The large number of cases requiring attendance every day only allowed hurried and imperfect examination. Often patients were detained in the waiting room for an inconvenient and 'injurious' length of time.[142] However,

Hodgkinson states that little further criticism was heard about the dispensary services after the middle of the nineteenth century.

The following table shows the large number of dispensaries that had been created in England and Wales by 1875. However, their distribution throughout the country was uneven, for instance Cambridge and Cardiff appear never to have had a free dispensary.

Table 15   Dispensaries in England and Wales 1875; details extracted from the 1875 *Medical Directory*[143].

County	Name	Established	Beds	Patients	Provident?
Bedfordshire-	Bedford Provident	1863			Yes
Berkshire	Christ's Hospital Abingdon	1862		660	
	Newbury	1835		1013	
	Reading	1802		8001	
	Sonning	1835		1200	
	Windsor Royal Disp and Infirmary	1818			
Buckinghamshire	High Wycombe Prov Disp	1884			Yes
Cambridgeshire	Ely	1862		320	
Cheshire	Altringcham	1870	12		
	Birkenhead Mission Disp	1866			
	Northwich	1871	8		
	Tranmere St Paul's Rd	1866		398	
	Ironbridge	1840			
	Stockport	1798			
	Wirral Hosp and Disp for sick children	1869	42		
Cornwall	East Cornwall	1844	16		
	Callington	1865		159	
	Cambourne Public	1842		170	
	Falmouth Public	1807		947	

	Helston Public	1809		220	
	Launceston Rowe	1862		260	
	Truro	1842		550	
	West Cornwall	1809	9		
Cumberland	Carlisle	1782		2719	
	Workington	1828		210	
Derbyshire	Bakewell Disp and Lying-In Institution	1830		450	
	Chesterfield and North Derbyshire	1855			
	Derby Provident Litchurch	1830		4843	Yes
Devonshire	Barnstaple and North Devon	1832		1291	
	Bideford Infirmary and Dispensary	1850	7		
	Dawlish	1855		350	
	Exeter	1818		4957	
	Exmouth	1868		514	
	Honiton	1820		270	
	Newton Cottage hosp and Dispensary	1858			
	Ottery St Mary Provident	1860		350	Yes
	Plymouth Provident			1050	Yes
	Plymouth Public	1798		3696	
	Sidmouth	1836		717	
	Tavistock	1832		511	
	Teignmouth, Dawlish and Newton Inf and Disp	1848	17		
	Tiverton Infirmary and Disp	1852			
	Torbay Hospital and Prov Disp	1844			Yes

Dorsetshire	Buckland Provident	1873		500
	Bridport Disp and cottage hospital	1867	8	
	Great Canford	1868		400
	Royal Portland	1840		240
Durham	Barnard Castle	1835		250
	Darlington Hospital and Disp	1809	19	
	Gateshead	1832		7616
	Hartlepools Hospital and Disp	1865	40	565
	Monkwearmouth and Southwick Disp	1873		
	South Shields and Westoe Disp	1821		4146
	Stockton-Upon-Tees	1863		1203
	Sunderland General Infirmary and Disp	1822	110	5672
Essex	Chelmsford Infirmary and Disp	1818	12	817
	Walthamstow	1873		870
Gloucestershire	Bristol Dispensary	1775		8403
	Bristol Eye Disp	1812		2000
	Cheltenham Coburg Soc and Disp for diseases of women and children	1817		200
	Cheltenham General Hosp and Disp	1839	90	6089
	Clifton Dispensary	1812		3153
	Clifton Disp for the cure of deafness	1851		180

	Frenchay General Disp	1819		347	
	Gloucester Prov Disp	1831		250	Yes
	Kingsdown Provident Disp Bristol	1870			Yes
	Minchinhampton			250	
	Redland General Disp for women and children and Disp for diseases of eye and ear Redland Branch Disp	1860		4000	
	Tetbury	1868		126	
	Tewkesbury	1815		422	
	Winterbourne General Disp	1819			
Hampshire	Bournemouth Gen Disp and cottage hosp	1859	6	1400	
	Ryde Disp	1849			
	Southampton Disp and Humane Soc	1823		3382	
	West Cowes			371	
Herefordshire	Hereford	1835		3156	
	Ledbury	1826		500	
	Leominster			599	
	Ross Disp and Cottage Hosp	1825	6	354	
	Yazor	1870		150	
Hertfordshire	St Alban's Hosp and Disp	1843	7	1112	
Kent	Belvedere	1855		198	
	Bexley	1866		300-500	
	Canterbury	1836		1870	
	Deal and Walmer	1862		540	
	Dover Hosp and Disp	1828		1602	
	Folkestone Disp and Infirmary	1846		618	

	Forest Hill	1865		1450	
	Gravesend and Milton Infirmary and Disp	1850	15	1496	
	Greenwich, Royal Kent Disp	1783		3810	
	Hythe	1849			
	Ramsgate and St Lawrence Royal Disp	1820		1550	
	Rochester, Chatham and Strood	1831		906	
	Sandgate	1844		94	
	Tunbridge Wells Disp and Infirmary	1828	38	4372	
Lancashire	Accrington and District	1874			
	Ashton-under-Lyme Provident Disp	1841			Yes
	Bolton Infirmary and Disp	1814	26	984	
	Bury General	1829		555	
	Chorley	1828		410	
	Garston Provident	1865			
	Hulme Disp Manchester			5736	
	Lancaster Infirmary and Disp	1731	70	3200	
	Liverpool	1778		65000	
	South Disp				
	North Disp				
	East Disp				
	Manchester Ardwick and Ancoats Hosp and Disp	1828	50	2766	
	Manchester Chorlton, Rusholme and Mossside Disp	1826			

128

	Manchester Clinical Hosp and Disp for children	1856	46	6073	
	Manchester Gen Hosp and Disp for sick children			8227	
	Manchester Medical Mission and Disp	1870		521	
	Manchester Royal Inf and Disp	1752	296	20916	
	Manchester Salford and Pendleton Royal Hosp and Disp	1828	60		
	Ormskirk	1797			
	Preston Amalgamated Friendly Socs Prov Disp	1870		3597	Yes
	Rochdale Infirmary and Disp	1832	8	739	
	Seaforth	1850	2	700	
	Southport Inf and local Dispensary	1827	20	1329	
	Warrington	1819		3000	
	Waterloo	1860		600	
	Wavertree, Childwell and Allerton	1819		200	
	Wigan Royal Albert Edward Inf and Disp	1798	60	4074	
	Woolton			500	
Leicestershire	Leicester Provident Disp	1862		15508	Yes
	Loughborough Inf and Disp	1819	20	1983	
	Market Harborough			314	
Lincolnshire	Boston Provident Disp	1852		3020	Yes
	Gainsborough	1828		500	

	Horncastle Public Disp	1789		763	
	Lincoln General Disp	1826		859	
	Louth Disp and Hospital	1803	20	907	
	Market Rasen Disp and Cottage Hosp	1856		152	
	Spalding Inf and Disp	1839		312	
Middlesex	Brentford	1818		260	
	Tottenham and Edmonton Gen Disp	1864		941	
Monmouthshire	Abergavenny	1828		632	
	Monmouth Gen Hosp and Dispensary	1810	10	1688	
	Newport Inf and Disp	1839	12	3590	
Norfolk	Norfolk and Norwich	1804		1647	
Northamptonshire	Royal Victoria Disp. Northampton	1844		15500	Yes
	Peterborough Inf and Disp and Fever Hosp	1815	42	3129	
Northumberland	Bamborough Casle	1772		1000	
	Berwick	1813		347	
	Hexham	1816		480	
	Morpeth	1816		518	
	Newcastle-upon-Tyne	1777		9417	
	Wooler Glendale	1824		240	
Nottinghamshire	Newark Hosp and Disp	1813	36	3579	
	Nottingham	1834		8035	
	East Retford	1865		700	
	Stapleford Village Infirmary and Disp	1865			

	Worksop General Disp	1867		822	
Oxfordshire	Oxford Medical Disp and Lying-in Charity	1807		1914	
Rutland	Rutland	1832		481	
Shropshire	Bridgnorth Infirmary and Disp	1841	8	729	
	Ironbridge	1828		1366	
	Ludlow			300-500	
	Oswestry	1828		1000	
	Shrewsbury	1843		1205	
	Wellington	1834		641	
	Wrockwardine and Eyton				
Somersetshire	Bath Disp and diseases of skin and urinary organs	1861		1000	
	Bath Eastern Disp	1832		3935	
	Bath Western Disp	1837		1168	
	Clevedon, Tickenham and Walton Disp	1843		1562	
	Frome St John's Disp	1854			
	Weston-super-Mare Hosp and Disp	1857	20	1256	
	Widcombe Southern Disp	1855		500	
Staffordshire	Burton-on-Trent Inf and Disp	1869	30	266	
	Lichfield	1781		923	
	Rugeley District Hosp and Prov Disp	1866	8	2178	Yes
Suffolk	Bungay Public Disp	1857		83	
	Lowestoft-Mutford and Lothi	1822		837	

Surrey	Southwold Disp	1837		162	
	Woodbridge-Seckforde	1861		395	
	Anerley Disp and Lying-in Charity	1864			
	Battersea	1845		650	
	Brixton, Streatham Hill	1850		3300	
	Camberwell Prov	1862			
	Charlwood Cottage Hosp and Disp	1873	4		
	Croydon	1835		700	
	Dulwich Prov Disp	1867		1500	Yes
	Kingston-on-Thames Prov	1865			Yes
	Norwood – Gypsey Hill and Upper Norwood	1868		3200	
	Penge General Disp and Lying-in Charity	1860		895	
	Richmond	1831		778	
	Surrey	1777		1230	
	Thames Ditton				
	Wandsworth Prov Disp	1862		3182	Yes
Sussex	Brighton and Hove	1809		8936	
	Brighton and Hove	1837		2215	
	Brighton –St John's, Carlton Hill	1870		2000	
	Chichester General Hosp and Disp	1827	60	1392	
	Eastbourne Prov Disp	1866		693	Yes
	East Grinstead Gen Disp	1858		700	
	Hastings	1830		1600	

	Lewes Infirmary and Disp	1847	3	936	
Warwickshire	Birmingham General Disp	1793		15896	
	Coventry Prov Disp	1831			Yes
	Erdington			215	
	Leamington Prov	1869		4000	Yes
	Warwick			2401	
Wiltshire	Devizes Cott Hosp and Disp	1872	6		
	North Wilts Disp	1860		308	
	Salisbury Prov Disp			4000	Yes
Worcestershire	Cookley and Wolverley	1834		1000	
	Dudley	1845		3661	
	Great Malvern	1830		907	
	Malvern Wells	1868		230	
	Stourbridge	1832		1215	
	Tenbury			300	
	Worcester Disp and Prov Medical Instituiton	1822		1840	Yes
Yorkshire	Barnsley	1865		2216	
	Beverley	1823		1678	
	Bradford Infirmary and Disp	1825	140	3480	
	Bridlington Cott Hosp and Disp	1868	6	187	
	Wakefield General Disp	1787	18	2934	
	Doncaster General Hosp and Disp	1792	24	2742	
	Hull and Sculcoates				
	Knaresborough				
	Leeds Public Disp	1824		23552	
	Leyburn				

	Malton	1830		140	
	Pontefract General Disp	1812		2280	
	Richmond	1835		126	
	Ripon	1840			
	Rotherham Hosp and Disp	1808	25	2800	
	Scarborough Disp and Accident Hosp	1852	3	1501	
	Sheffield Public Hosp and Disp	1832	104	27145	
	Whitby Public Disp	1786		600	
	York	1788		4665	
Carnarvonshire	Carnarvonshire and Anglesey Inf and Disp	1845	20	1696	
Denbighshire	Denbighshire Inf and Gen Disp	1807	40	3120	
	Wrexham Inf and General Disp	1833	30	2096	
Flintshire	Flintshire	1824		1600	
Glamorganshire	Cardiff Inf and Disp	1836	52	3357	
Montgomeryshire	Welshpool	1827		566	
Pembrokeshire	Pembroke Disp and Inf	1862	8	217	
Isle of Man	Isle of Man Gen Hosp and Disp	1839	32	1090	
London	Bloomsbury Disp	1801			
	Camden and Kentish Towns Prov D	1871		300	Yes
	Central Pancras Prov Disp	1854			Yes
	Chelsea, Brompton and Belgrave D	1812		6029	
	Child's Hill Prov Disp	1872			Yes

Chiswick and Turnham Green	1853	633	
City Disp	1789	16825	
City of London and East London Disp	1849	14000	
Clapham General Disp	1849		
Dulwich Prov Disp	1867	1500	Yes
Eastern Dispensay W	1782	3262	
Faringdon General Disp	1828	20004	
Finsbury	1780	9626	
French Hospital and Disp	1867	20	
Hampstead Prov Disp	1845	1333	Yes
Haverstock Hill and Malden Rd Prov D	1865	2403	Yes
Hendon Prov Disp			Yes
Highgate	1787	1090	
Holloway and N Islington Disp	1840	9179	
Islington	1821	9295	
Islington and N London Prov Disp	1864		Yes
Kensington	1840	5499	
Kilburn, Maida Vale and St John Gen D	1862	8017	
London Disp	1777	3273	
London Medical Mission Disp	1871	6100	
Metropolitan Disp	1797	10000	
North West London Free Disp for sick children			
Nottinghill Prov Disp	1860		Yes

Paddington Prov Disp	1837	6366	Yes
Plumstead	1864	300	
Portland Town Free Disp	1845		
Public Disp for relief of sick poor	1782	4000	
Queen Adelaide's Disp	1850	43088	
Royal Disp for diseases of ear			
Royal General Dispensary	1770	1600	
Royal Pimlico D and Lying-in Charity	1831	9000	
Royal South London Disp			
St George's and St James Disp	1817	6962	
St James's and St Anne's Disp	1858	7095	
Royal Kent Disp Greenwich	1783	3810	
Royal Pimlico Disp and lying-in charity	1831	9000	
Royal South London Disp			
St Anne's disp, Stamford hill	1872		
St George's (Hanover Sq) Prov Disp	1868		Yes
St George's and St James Disp	1858	7095	
St John's wood and Portland Town Prov	1845	2516	Yes
St Marylebone General Disp	1785		
St Marylebone Prov Disp	1836	3500	Yes
St Pancras and Northern Disp	1810	4452	

St Paul's and St Barnabas Disp	1810	4452	
City Provident Disp for diseases of skin	1865	3000	Yes
South Lambeth, Stockwell, North Brixton	1866	2572	
Stamford Hill, Stoke Newington etc	1825		
Surrey	1777	1230	
Tower Hamlets	1792	2569	
Walworth Provident Disp	1870	6500	Yes
Wandsworth Prov Disp	1862	3182	Yes
Westbourne Prov Disp and maternity	1856		Yes
Western City Disp			
Western Disp Broadway, Westminster			
Western Disp for diseases of skin			
Western General Disp Marylebone rd	1830	5468	
Westminster General Disp	1774	9771	
South London Dispensary for women and children	30	1000	

Selected Provincial Dispensaries

The Stroud Dispensary—The First Provincial Dispensary

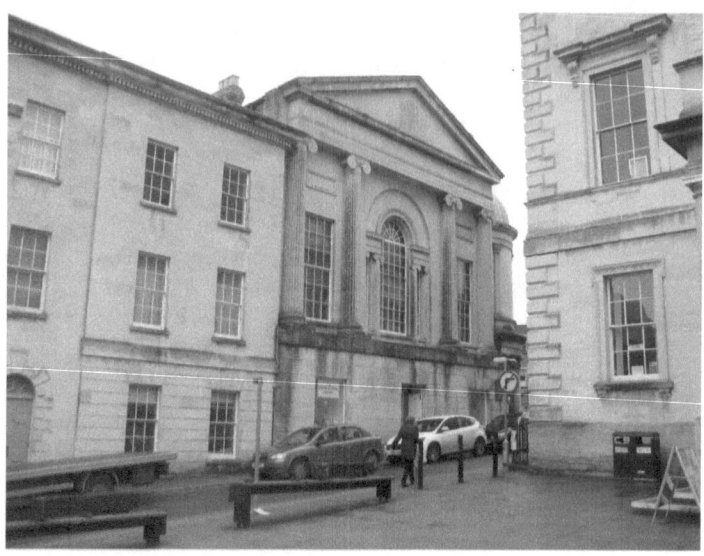

The dispensary and casualty ward to the left of
the subscription rooms, Stroud, 2015.

Stroud, a town in Gloucestershire, has the distinction of having
had the first provincial dispensary in England. Stroud was involved
in an early Industrial Revolution based on the cloth trade, and in 1754
it was claimed that the town was the most populous spot of ground
in the three kingdoms.[144] In 1755 the 'dispensatory' was described as
a 'laudable scheme' to support and relieve the poor 'in their state of
sickness and consequent distress' and had already established a good
reputation. The dispensary, funded by annual subscriptions, provided
free medicines and medical advice to the poor of Stroud.[145] In 1771
Dr Samuel Jones, the physician, wrote the prescriptions and kept the
accounts. Mr Thomas Hughes was the apothecary (for twenty-five
years), who dispensed the medicines – he was very knowledgeable,
highly regarded, and was a surgeon and man-midwife. From 1782–3
the dispensary treated 774 patients, of whom 355 were cured, 6 were

incurable, 18 died, and the rest improved. This cost £570, received in subscriptions.

In January 1784, for each guinea paid annually, the subscribers were entitled to send one person a week for treatment. However, by May, the demand had increased, they were running into debt, and the number of patients had to be restricted to six patients a year per guinea. There was more sickness amongst the poor, who were 'in distress' due to the decline in the clothing trade, partly owing to 'the American war'. For the year of 1785 Mr Hughes was paid £30 for dispensing the medicines, but he would only accept £25. The drug bill was £37. 9 shillings, sundries £12, and rent and coal for the physician's room came to £2. 9 shillings.

The patients saw the physician in a single hired room – at Mr Mills's cottage in Wallbridge for three years; then at the Lamb Inn, Church Street for six years; and then adjoining the King's Arms for twelve years. The patients then had to wait outside Mr Hughes's house on High Street while he dispensed the medicines. Eventually, in 1805, rooms were rented at Richard Playne's house in Rowcroft to include a waiting room for the patients. By 1823 the society had enough funds to buy a plot of land in Kendrick's Orchard and build their own dispensary. It cost a total of £741 11s 10d and formed the angle between the new streets (that were later to be called George Street and Bedford Street). A casualty ward was provided by adding a stone building next door to the brick dispensary in 1835. It cost £308 7s, and the ward paid an annual rent of £16 to the dispensary. It had a surgeon and a nurse and was for 'persons who might meet with accidental injuries, requiring immediate surgical aid in order to avoid exposing them to the painful and dangerous journey to the Infirmary at Gloucester'. In 1859 the dispensary and Casualty Hospital were renamed Stroud General Hospital.

The Warrington Dispensary[146]

Most dispensaries had few academic links or aspirations, but this was not the case with the Warrington Dispensary. The dispensary was established in 1810 by Dr James Kendrick. It had two local Members of Parliament on its inaugurating committee and soon occupied a medium sized three-storey Georgian building in one of Warrington's main streets. Kendrick was born in 1770, was apprenticed to a local apothecary, and went on to practise there until he died at the age of 76. To his successful practice he added a fellowship of the Linnaean Society and published medical treatises of his own; he edited many others through a close association with the local printing house of Eyres, which had been associated with the Warrington Academy. Kendrick's taste for academic activities had been encouraged by the atmosphere he had been brought up in association with the Warrington Academy, and the dispensary developed a literary and scientific society, at which papers were read and where the local medical apprentices were encouraged to attend. A library was housed in the committee room. The first printed catalogue of the library is dated 1834. It is prefaced by the rules which show there was an obligation on the librarian (the resident apothecary for the time being) to replace all lost books at his own expense. It was also stated that the circulating membership was to extend beyond the town and that the annual subscription was to be one guinea. Two apprentices were attached to the dispensary and their indenture fees of £25 were also allocated to the library funds. It was estimated that this, together with the subscriptions, would give them about £20 a year to spend on books.

The Warrington Dispensary Library remained in active use until its removal to a new building in 1874. It was then that the books were put in a loft to be left as lumber for thirty-five years, their value to the medical historian unrecognised except to the firm of booksellers in the town who had been associated with its collection from the start. It was they, no doubt, who got in touch with Sawyers of London from whom William Osler bought the complete set in 1907 and took it to America to contribute to the Johns Hopkins University medical library.

The Whitehaven Dispensary[147]

Whitehaven is a small seaside town to the west of the Lake district. Around 1750 it had a thriving port exporting coal and importing tobacco. This dispensary was promoted by local physician Dr Joshua Dixon and was opened in 1783 on Scotch Street. In its first year 1,467 patients were recommended and registered. There were also 433 trivial cases, and 157 children were treated for smallpox. Of the 1,467 patients, 1,089 were cured, 110 died, and 1,021 were attended in their own homes. The diseases were as listed in table 16:

Table 16   The diseases treated at the Whitehaven Dispensary 1783

Disease	Number of cases	Disease	Number of cases
Intermittent fever	9	Flatulence	42
Inflammatory fever	55	Convulsions	4
Hectic fever	4	Epilepsy	9
Worm fever	84	Asthma	29
External inflammation	25	Whooping cough	24
Inflammation of eyes	27	Colic	47
Inflammation of brain	1	Diarrhoea	25
Inflammation of forethroat	12	Hysteria	4
Inflammation of lungs	51	Melancholy	2
Inflammation of bowels	1	Chronic weakness	22
Acute rheumatism	16	Dropsy	15
Chronic rheumatism	29	Rickets	5
Erisipelas	8	Scrophula	20

Inflammation eruptions	15	Lues venerea	7
Natural smallpox	320	Jaundice	4
Inoculated smallpox	30	Dimness of sight	8
Miliary fever	2	Deafness	2
Haemorrhages	17	Gravel	13
Consumption	37	Aneurysm	1
Abortion	1	Schirrus	2
Catarrh	35	Cancer	4
Catarrh of old age	7	Rupture	2
Dysentery	49	Scald head	9
Headache and vertigo	32	White swelling	2
Palsy	6	Scorbutic eruptions	98
Fainting	3	Luxations, fractures etc	18
Stomach complaints	46	Ulcers and abscesses	42
Contusions, wounds, etc	58		
		Total	1467

During the first year of the dispensary, from June 1783 until June 1784, 1,467 patients were seen by letter of recommendation. In addition, 433 patients presented themselves to the dispensary without any recommendation and were classed as 'trivial cases' and seen by the apothecary. One thousand twenty-one of the recommended cases were visited in their own homes by the apothecary William Robinson, who was given a gratuity of five guineas for the work he had done in addition to his £30 a year salary.

Loudon[148] compared the costs of several of the dispensaries showing how inexpensive Whitehaven Dispensary was:

Table 17   Comparison of the Costs of various dispensaries

Institution	Year	Expenditure £	Outpatients	Total admissions	Cost per admission
Surrey Dispensary	1785	1019	4689	4689	4s 4d
Liverpool Dispensary	1810	1494	1004	10408	2s 10d
Newcastle Dispensary	1802	3311	3017	3017	3s 1d
Carlisle Dispensary	1800	345	3143	3143	2s 2d
Whitehaven Dispensary	1799	157	4964	4964	0s 7½d

The Liverpool Dispensaries

The first Liverpool Dispensary was founded in 1778 at the annual vestry of the parishioners of the Parish of Liverpool, where it was decided to pay an annual sum of 100 guineas to fund the dispensary, instead of paying for the services of an apothecary.[149] These annual parish grants continued until 1840, after which the dispensary became totally dependent on public contributions. This original dispensary opened at 25 Princes Street with three surgeons, three physicians, and an apothecary/secretary, and in the first year 2,062 patients were treated. The next year the dispensary took over the medical work at the Blue Coat School and the gaol, and 7,348 patients were treated. In 1782 the dispensary moved into a purpose-built premises on the corner of Church Street and Old Post Office Place, and it was arranged for the dispensary to further extend its role with caring for the seaman's hospital and the alms houses, the workhouse, the house of correction, the fever recovery hospital, and the lunatic asylum! With the volume of work still increasing, it was decided to operate on a regional basis. In 1824 the South Dispensary in Upper Parliament Street was opened. In 1831 the North Dispensary in Vauxhall Road was built, and the site on Church Street was sold for £6000.

The annual report of the Liverpool Dispensaries of 1838 tells of increasing financial difficulties.[150] These were put down to the agreement to include the townships of Everton and Kirkdale within the area of the dispensaries' work, the immense advance in the price of leeches, and various alterations in the North and South dispensaries. The number of patients treated during the year was 42,239. The rules of the institution give a clear indication of the workload of the staff and committee members. The general committee met once a month, and the subcommittee responsible for each dispensary met each week to order medicines, instruments, and furniture and to examine the situation and wants of the institution. The combined post of secretary and collector of subscriptions was full-time and salaried. Physicians and surgeons were elected by ballot, constituted the medical board, and met monthly. The honorary physician and surgeon attended the dispensary every day (except Sundays) at 10 a.m., followed by home visiting. Apparently no amputations or other important operations were allowed without consultations with two honorary surgeons.

Salaried house surgeons were attached to each dispensary and had to devote all their time to the job. They had to keep the records and registers and were expected to be in attendance most of the time. There was also an assistant house physician in residence who had a district allocated to him. He was expected to start to visit his patients no later than 10.30 a.m. and to return by 3 p.m. when he was on duty in the dispensary.

There were also apprentices who paid 100 guineas as an admission fee, were in post for five years, and paid 20 guineas a year for the privilege. They were examined every six months by the medical board who reported on their progress. The honorary medical officers also had their pupils at the dispensary for short periods.

The gratuitous work of the honorary physicians and surgeons caused some discontent and a distinguished Liverpool physician, John Rutter, who had worked in a dispensary for thirteen years, addressed the local doctors:[151]

In this place you [doctors] may be able sooner or later, to originate measures which may terminate in procuring for all who are engaged in the service of our public institutions, a fair and just remuneration for their labours.... Some time must elapse before you can prevail on the inhabitants of Liverpool to think that it is neither just not reasonable that so many of you should be expected to employ the best and most active period of your life in labouring for the public without reward. Unrewarded duties and services such as yours, so extensive, and so unremitting, have not yet been expected from any other portion of the community, and ought not to be expected from you.

The number of patients attended by Poor Law doctors in Liverpool was trifling when compared with those receiving relief from the dispensaries, and to add insult to injury, the dispensary honorary medical officers were expected to attend patients in the workhouse and the fever hospital for no remuneration, whereas the Poor Law doctors received a salary. The withdrawal of the parish donation to the Liverpool dispensaries as a result of the need to pay the Poor Law doctors caused major problems to the Liverpool dispensaries, and in 1844 Dr HW Rumsey told the select committee on the Poor Laws that 'notwithstanding that the dispensaries relieve them of the expenditure of several thousand a year, which but for these institutions would fall on the town at large in the shape of additional poor rates'.

Another organisation had started the St Anne's Dispensary in Islington in 1839, but this work was soon taken over by the committee of the dispensaries, who transferred the work to a new building in Richmond Row in 1865, calling it the East Dispensary. This was completely rebuilt in 1910.

In 1934, to serve the needs of the new housing area in Huyton, a temporary branch was opened. In 1940 this was replaced with a purpose-built modern dispensary. In 1935 the four dispensaries coped with 103,968 attendances from 20,609 patients.

The dispensary service was completely free until about 1830, when financial difficulties forced the committee to make a charge of one penny for each attendance and also to pay another penny for any tooth extraction that was necessary. Gradually the fee was increased in 1940 to 6d for adults and 6d for children.

The committee report for 1875 described the high numbers of patients who had been relieved in the previous year:

North Dispensary   23,765   South Dispensary   18,828
East Dispensary   25,484

Many of the patients were found in utterly destitute circumstances and may have had to be transferred to the care of parish authorities.

One of the former house surgeons of one of the Liverpool dispensaries, Michael Robert Sheridan, who became an ear nose and throat surgeon in Truro, wrote in 1978 of his experience as a dispensary doctor around 1930[152]:

> The city council made the appointments, and the salary in those days was £200 per annum, (I am almost certain), which even in those days, for a total commitment, was hardly generous. Each appointed doctor had his 'district', which was blocks of streets. We had responsibility for several streets near Boundary Street and extending up to the Stanley Hospital area. The dispensary surgery was held daily in a street off Stanley Road. There, in a biggish room, from 11 a.m. on to 12.30 or later I saw maybe twenty patients. Within a few feet of me was Dr Robinson, separated by a thin six-foot partition with his patients from an adjoining district. Behind both of us was the dispenser, Mr Pugh, a good man. He had a chest with several made-up mixtures, which simply needed

dilution. There were also tablets, etc. The thing most coveted by the patients was cod liver oil and malt!

The noise amounted to several decibels, but nobody seemed to mind and nothing very intimate was complained of. Most of the patients were mothers and babies, who quite often came for treatment for both of them. Babies had mainly diarrhoea and vomiting or bronchitis. Mothers had coughs, etc. There was a couch and screen for examining chests and abdomens, etc. Chest exams were often rather cursory! I doubt whether our drugs did much good. At least they had none of the side effect of some modern drugs.

Record keeping was minimal. Each patient brought a prescription sheet, and they were entered in a book with a diagnosis. Each was given another appointment if necessary. Request for visits were supposed to be handed in at the surgery; they would be fulfilled in the afternoons. No charges were made for anything. Requests for emergency visits often came in the evening and had to have the sanction of the Relieving Officer. The houses the patients had were very poor and, often, I fear, smelly and dirty. The patients were very poor. We had few adult male patients as they had panel doctors, but if unemployed and 'ceased insurance', they became parish patients. Pneumonia and bronchopneumonia were dreaded things, and here the district nurse could be called in for support. Poverty, in those days, really was abject, as you will remember.

In the end the work got me down, and I was glad to make the change.

The Nottingham Dispensary[153]

The Nottingham General Hospital was one of the last voluntary hospitals to open its doors to patients, in 1782. Similarly, the Nottingham Dispensary was established quite late in the dispensary movement, opening only on 9 May 1831. A letter from eighty inhabitants to the local press on 16 December 1830 called for the establishment of a dispensary, as the hospital was finding it impossible to cope with large numbers of outpatients. The original proposal was to have the dispensary annexed to the Hospital and that their funds should be shared.[154] However, this proposal was rejected by the governors.

The new dispensary was created in a large house situated between Hockley and Woolpack Lane at a yearly rent of £35. The 'founding fathers' included the Duke of Newcastle as president, leading bankers, senior clergy, and numerous civic dignitaries, including the current and future mayors.

There was much competition to become honorary physicians and surgeons. The resident surgeon and apothecary was Mr Robert Garner until May 1832. After that Mr Isaac Massey was appointed, and he continued until 1836. The main committee appointed subcommittees with specialist members to investigate, check, control, and recommend action in specific areas. The finance committee inspected and controlled the maintenance and repairs of all medical and household equipment and the fabric of the dispensary's buildings. The drug committee, with its medical members' and dispensers' views to call on, controlled the selection of drugs used by the dispensary and recommended the policy on sourcing supply. In 1855 there was a debate as to whether to continue to source on a quarterly basis from Nottingham druggists or whether for cost-benefit reasons to source from London wholesalers. At the meeting on 16 July, Dr Massey's views prevailed and a compromise was reached to take the supply of the main items from London and the rest from local druggists.

The drug committee also kept an eye on drug costs. An investigation in 1899 looked into the excessive cost of drugs used at the Hyson Green branch, which were twice that of Broad Street. The drug committee report stated

1. there must be either a. extravagance in prescribing; b. extravagance in dispensing; c. absolute waste; d. systematic robbery; or e. a combination of the latter three;
2. to direct the branch doctor's serious attention to the matter and ask him to supervise ordering of the drugs and surgical dressings for the branch;
3. to serve notice on Dispenser Coates (of the Hyson Green branch) and engage a new full-time dispenser at £90 per annum;
4. all drugs and surgical dressings for the branch to be ordered through Broad Street except for emergencies. London drugs to go through Broad Street;
5. Smithurst (the Broad Street Dispenser) should take stock at the branch, and superfluous quantities should be returned.

The excessive drugs bill for the branch had in fact been caused by the corrupt actions of Dispenser Coates. All supplies came from his own druggist business and none from a London source.

From the start the dispensary operated on a recommendation with donors and subscribers having privileges. Rule 3 stated 'Donors of £5.5.0 or subscribers of 10s 6d shall have the privilege of recommending three patients; donors of £10.10.0 or subscribers of £1.0.0 recommend six patients. Donors of £21 or subscribers of £2.2.0 recommend twelve patients, and in the same proportion for any higher donation or subscription. Rule 4 indicated 'a recommendation for a patient to be visited at home is equivalent to two recommendations for patients personally attending the dispensary and a recommendation for a truss equal to three recommendations'.

Rule 6 stated 'donors of £10.10.0 or subscribers of £1.1.0 and upwards are governors.

Rule 7 stated 'Ministers preaching sermons and making collections for the benefit of the charity, or the individual paying in money so collected, are considered as contributing subscriptions and have the privilege of recommending patients in proportion to the sums which they shall respectively pay into the hands of the treasurers'. The incentive of recommendation was also given to the local government body, which from time to time sought medical assistance from the dispensary especially in times of epidemics, and to Friendly Societies seeking treatment for members.

Rule 8 stated 'the Chief Magistrate of anybody corporate given a subscription, or the person appointed by any society to pay a subscription, shall have the same power of recommending patients as a subscriber'. Special rights were given to the honorary medical officers.

Rule 13 stated 'The physicians and surgeons giving their professional gratuitous services to the institution are governors and each of them during their attendance shall exercise the same privilege as subscribers of £5.5.0'.

In 1888 donor privileges were halved in an attempt to exercise some control over the growing patient numbers. The rules required each honorary physician to be consulted at the dispensary 'in weekly rotation'. Each honorary surgeon had to attend the dispensary to advise his patients at 10 a.m. two days per week on a rotating basis. Honorary medical officers from 1850 onwards had to have resided or practised in Nottingham for at least one year preceding the day of their election.

Unusually, after the first twenty-eight years of the dispensary's operation, the honorary medical officers started receiving fees for the first time in 1859. The fees were fixed and regulated by the committee. The amount to be paid to the doctors was only £1 per week, but there was much controversy, and many subscribers were unhappy with these payments. In 1864 the honorary medical officers agreed to give up their fees so that the money could be spent on appointing a much-needed assistant resident surgeon. Thereafter, as in the great majority of other dispensaries, the honorary medical officers received no fees or salary.

Each resident medical officer (RMO) was appointed for three years until 1902 when the engagement period was reduced to two as it was becoming more difficult to recruit resident surgeons. These RMOs were not allowed to have any other professional business. As well as his annual salary the resident surgeon and apothecary 'shall have the benefit of the house, clear of all outgoings of rent, taxes, and rates; coals and candles'. He had to 'cause the medicines duly to be compounded in conformity with the prescriptions and directions of the medical offices, and cause them to be delivered, properly labelled, with plain and accurate directions to the patients'.

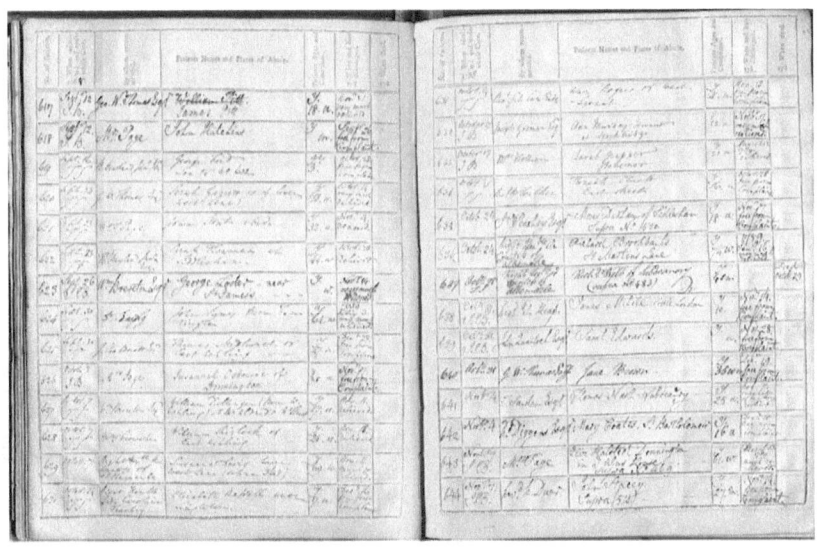

Day book from the Chichester Dispensary from the late eighteenth century. Courtesy West Sussex Record Office.

The resident surgeon was obliged to register the names, ages, residences, and diseases of the patients, distinguishing those who attend the dispensary from those who were attended at their own homes, and stated when each was admitted, by whom recommended, by whom attended, when discharged, and in what state. He performed minor operations of surgery at the desire of the surgeons and caused the general dressings for the surgical patients to be prepared every morning and kept in readiness. He also had to keep an inventory of surgical instruments. He had to report to the committee 'if from appearances it looks as if the patient could pay'. He constantly endeavoured to use the most rigid economy in the consumption of drugs and other articles and not to give orders for any, excepting by the directions of the committee.

The working days were long at the dispensary. It opened every day except Sunday at 9 a.m. and closed at 10 p.m.; but medicine prescribed in the course of the day need not be delivered after seven o'clock, except in cases of emergency. Resident surgeons could be local or from anywhere in Britain. Posts were advertised locally and from 1823 in *The Lancet* and from 1858 in the *British Medical Journal.*

In 1857 there were subscriber complaints against the honorary medical officers accusing them of not being as attentive to patients as they ought to be. The inference throughout the committee minutes is that in many situations the resident medical staff thought they were competent themselves to deal with most cases and did not have much need of the honorary medical staff.

In 1863 it was stated that the house surgeon's work had doubled since 1832 (from 443 to 843 home visits). On Mondays he had, during the busy portion of the year, to see as many as 60 or 70 patients, at their respective homes in the course of the day; and on average, throughout the week he had to attend to 74 out and home patients daily.... In addition, since enclosure (1845) to the North and South sides of the town inhabited portions of the borough have greatly extended ... (to) over three times the area the dispensary covered in 1831. Already these distant cases grew from 19 in 1855 to 181 in 1863.

Table 18   Workload of the Nottingham Dispensary

Year	Home Patients	Per cent of total patients
1831	443	17.31
1841	1104	34.88
1851	1209	33.8
1861	1081	11.01

1871	1131	14.19
1881	1274	14.7
1891	1308	15
1901	1497	12.1
1911	1589	9.47

The types of accidents and emergencies dealt with by the Dispensary in 1851

Fractures of upper extremities 126, or lower 115	241
Injuries of upper extremities 424, of lower 235	659
Burns 186, Abscesses opening 35, diseases of urinary organs	308
Intestinal ruptures 26, Froenum Linguae 32, Diarrhoea 192	250
Organs of respiration 92, of circulation 4, of digestion 51	147
Measles, scarlatina, fever, erysipelas	53
Cases of poisoning 15, Hysteria 14, Ophthalmia 3, Haemorrhage	37
Others	47
Total	1642

Teeth extraction formed part of the routine work of RMOs at the dispensary, and a honorary dental surgeon was appointed in 1867.

The growth in patient numbers meant that in fewer than ten years, the dispensary had outgrown the premises in Hockley. In response to this situation, a purpose-built premises was constructed in Broad Street at a cost of £1797 opening in 1841. The new building was designed to demonstrate to the outside world the munificence of the supporters of the charity and to be an object of civic pride. A two-floored building was stuccoed and had Grecian columns. Major improvements were made in 1859 when a new waiting room, consulting room, and operating room were opened. An additional surgeon was appointed April 1864 and another in 1882 when accommodation in the dispensary was increased. In 1896 a branch dispensary was opened at 130 Gregory Boulevard, Hyson Green. In 1899 the city was divided into four districts for home visiting purposes, with two surgeons to each building.

Table 19   Number of patients seen in the Nottingham dispensaries 1897-1911

Numbers of patients

1897		Broad St	Hyson Green	Total
	Home	1507	257	1764
	Out	8878	1672	10554
	Dental	1690	497	2187
				14501
1900	Home	1219	256	1475
	Out	6126	3035	9161
	Dental	1419	1612	3031
				13667
1911	Home	1049	540	1589
	Out	7406	4434	11840
	Dental	2111	1247	3358
				16787

In 1840 the dispensary decided to stop midwifery care. Up to that year it had provided medical attendance as well as a midwife.

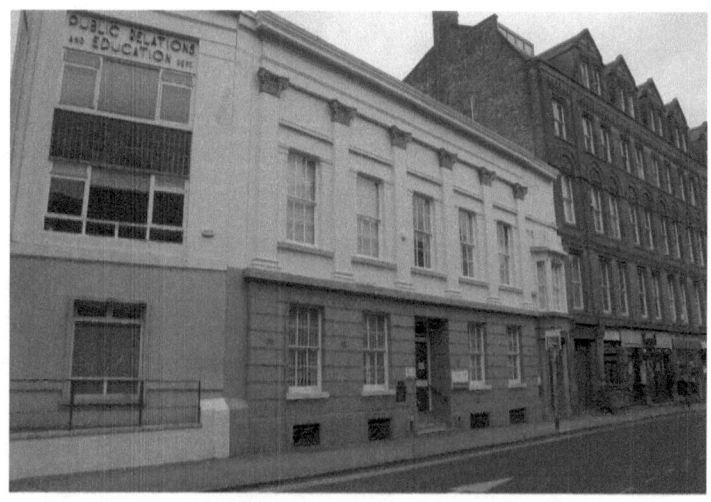

The Nottingham Dispensary, courtesy 'Jonfholl' via Flikr.com.
Built 1841, with the bay on the extreme right added 1883.

The governors considered introducing a provident system, and in 1872 a deputation from the committee was delegated to study the provident system in Leicester. In the annual report of that year the decision was reported that they were reluctant to move from being a free charity and preferred to solicit funds from other sources such as from operatives and employers. The Hospital Sunday and Saturday funds were set up primarily to aid the finances of the General Hospital and only secondarily to give some modest support to the dispensary and other medical charities. The dispensary was always dissatisfied with the small sums it received from the two funds, and this was expressed in a number of annual reports (e.g., see the reports from 1873 and 1875). Apprentice fees provided some income although it was sporadic. The 1845 annual report contained a typical advertisement: 'Institution in want of an apprentice – premium £150'.

John Smithurst, the future dispenser, was engaged as an apprentice. His father paid a £50 premium at the time of binding, £50 more six months later, and another £50 at the end of twelve months. The apprenticeship lasted five years.

Earnings from dividends and interest became the second most important source of Income for the dispensary – second to the subscriptions.

Table 20   Income of the Nottingham Dispensary

Year	Total income £	Subscriptions £	Subscriptions as per cent of total income
1831	1300	574	44.15
1851	620	453	73.11
1871	1272	655	51.53
1891	1777	927	52.19
1911	4274	1565	36.63

The Ancoats Dispensary, Manchester

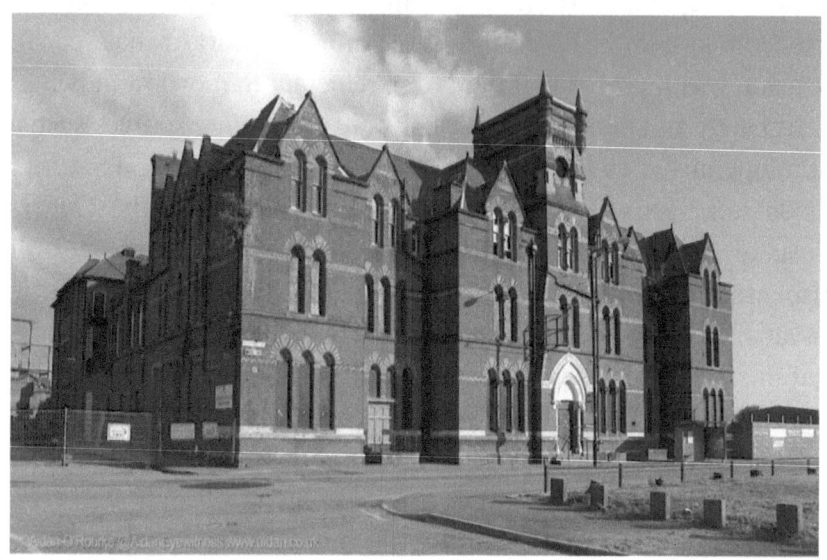

Courtesy Aiden O'Rourke
This dispensary is the only one that I have discovered to be
well-known in the twenty-first century, for it is the subject
of considerable media attention as it has attracted large
local and national support for a re-building project.[155]

Ancoats Dispensary was one of several in Manchester and was the
third to be opened, on 11 August 1828, and was formed to provide
free medical care for the poor in the suburb of Ancoats. These
included the many factory workers in the numerous cotton mills, the
handloom weavers, and the labourers. The dispensary was funded by
the wealthy owners of the local industries and was intended to help
relieve the overburdened Manchester Infirmary. The predecessors
of the Ancoats Dispensary were the one at Chorlton-on-Medlock
(formed in 1825) and Salford and Pendleton (formed in 1827).

The dispensary's first president was George Murray, the owner
of a large textile mill complex in the area and the first physician. One
of the other founders was Dr James Kay, who wrote the small book
Moral and Physical Condition of the Working Classes (1832) based
on his experiences in the dispensary. He drew attention to the fact

that charity tended to promote poverty rather than help relieve it. By July 1833 the dispensary had treated more than thirteen thousand people stricken mostly with accidents and infectious diseases.

The dispensary moved to Ancoats Crescent in 1850 and to 94 Mill Street in 1869. A further move to larger premises on Mill Street was followed by a gift from Hannah Brackenbury. The funds were further supported by local workers who set up a Workpeople's Fund Committee and ensured that the institution was without debt for the first time in its history. In 1879 the dispensary opened six beds and it was at this time that the organisation became known officially as 'Ancoats Hospital and Ardwick and Ancoats Dispensary', although this was generally shortened to Ancoats Hospital.

Originally, the building had three storeys above basement level and it is probable that the ground floor accommodated the physicians' entrance, patient entrance, and waiting rooms, sitting rooms, dispensing room, and consulting rooms, with the upper floors accommodating board, room, offices, library, private rooms, and wards.

The dispensary function of the hospital became a provident dispensary in 1875; the management of this was transferred to the Manchester and Salford Provident Dispensaries Association in 1885. Means testing was introduced by the association, which had arrangements with hospitals for the provision of treatment, midwifery services, and similar requirements as well as providing care itself for, at worst, a minimal charge. People were eligible for membership if they were unable to obtain poor relief but too impoverished to afford medical care. The members paid a joining fee and a regular subscription. An extension to the hospital was completed in 1888, providing an additional fifty beds and a further fourteen by 1915. A rural convalescent home opened near Alderley Edge in 1904.

Throughout its existence, the dispensary and hospital always had to struggle to fund itself, but in spite of this was able to provide the city's first x-ray department in 1907. In 1914 Harry Platt – who was later to become well-known orthopaedic surgeon – started the world's first fracture clinic. Platt also introduced physiotherapy facilities in 1920.

The Huddersfield Dispensary

Nineteenth-century Huddersfield in the West Riding of Yorkshire was a town of about thirteen thousand in 1821 and was experiencing the typical expansion of the Industrial Revolution based on the textile industry. In 1814 the dispensary became the first charity of any significance to be set up in Huddersfield.[156] The officers and committee members were mostly local merchants and manufacturers. Unusually, there were no members of the local gentry, clergymen, doctors, lawyers, or bankers on the organising committee. The main motives behind the creation of the dispensary appeared to be to provide a cheap and efficient form of medical relief for cases among the sick poor, particularly accidents as a result of manufacturing processes, and infectious diseases that threatened to invade the homes of the wealthy, avoiding the likely financial burdens on the ratepayers and employers.

A purpose-built Infirmary was established in connection with the dispensary in 1831, and in 1865 the support of both the dispensary and Infirmary continued to be largely from the manufacturing and marketing of textiles. Fifty-three per cent of the subscribers that year were merchants and manufacturers, 24 per cent were tradesman, and the remainder were gentlemen, clergy, and farmers.

The Infirmary's main function was to look after large numbers of accident patients, the only category that could be admitted directly without a subscriber's recommendation. In 1846, 379 accident cases were admitted, and these often made up the majority of inpatient admissions. In 1861 there were 3,787 outpatients and 176 inpatients, and this ratio of 22:1 was not atypical. In that year almost 11 per cent of the inhabitants of Huddersfield had received dispensary treatment, compared with 0.5 per cent admitted as inpatients. In 1838 the great majority of inpatients were 60 years of age or younger – only 4 per cent were older than that age.

For a doctor to obtain an honorary post attached to the Infirmary or dispensary, he would have to be in something of an elite position in the local medical and social hierarchy. An honorary appointee would preferably be Huddersfield born and raised, at best a member of a medical dynasty, but, if not, of a sound family background.[157] Most honorary medical officers retained their posts for many years, some for between forty and sixty years!

As in other towns and cities there was an attempt to introduce a provident system. In 1859 Samuel Knaggs, a Huddersfield general practitioner, and a strong advocate of self-help dispensaries and insurance societies, proposed setting up a self-help medical provision for the poor of the town as an alternative to medical charity. Knagg's suggestion to the Infirmary was rejected out of hand, and a few years later, in 1863, he overcame his scruples, being appointed honorary surgeon!

The Warwick Dispensary

The Warwick Dispensary, 1826–70,[158] was established in March 1826 by a group of local notables, 'for the relief of the sick and necessitous poor of the borough and its vicinity'. The context of need arose both from national economic depression and local distress, various textile mills having closed after a brief boom. The Earl of Warwick and Chandos Leigh of Stoneleigh were invited to become patron and president respectively, while the seven vice presidents included five Warwickshire members of parliament. The forty-three initial subscribers were divided roughly equally between similar 'county' figures and prominent local business and professional people. They included the surgeon Henry Lilley Smith, who in 1823 had founded the first provident or 'self-supporting' dispensary in nearby Southam. However, the new institution was established on the more familiar, purely charitable lines.

Its income was based on subscriptions and donations from the affluent as well as an annual ball; the subscribers (or governors) elected the committee and were entitled to issue letters of recommendation for treatment in proportion to the sum subscribed. Of the 137 subscribers in 1869, about half were either titled or 'gentry', rather broadly defined. The clearly needy were those eligible to receive gratuitous treatment as 'free members', but exact criteria are unclear. Two physicians, four surgeons, and a dispenser were appointed to attend patients twice weekly at the dispensary or at their homes, initially using a house in the High Street. In 1843 the committee purchased 8 Castle Street. Unusually, the medical men were paid 5s per case, from which they could earn up to £60 annually. The physicians appear to have participated fully in the rosters with the surgeons rather than acting purely as consultants. The number of patients treated increased over time; 278 were admitted in the second year of operation (March 1827–8). In 1856–7, 391 new patients were treated. In 1868 the rules were altered to allow free choice of medical attendant and an increased number of tickets for subscribers. By 1869–70, the levels of demand, with 841 new patients that year, were causing such financial strain that the committee decided to explore alternative approaches to funding.

Royal Portland Dispensary[159]

This dispensary, despite its royal patronage, had no premises and was unique in the way it was run. The dispensary was founded by the quarry owners and principal stone merchants to afford relief to their quarry workers with large families, especially in times when the trade of the island was fluctuating and the men were working on short time. It was established in 1840 under the direct patronage of Queen Victoria who contributed £25 a year to the charity throughout her reign. Her link to the dispensary was probably through Prince Albert, who had taken a major interest in the development of the naval dockyard at Portland.

In 1899 the two doctors, Henley and Lawson, received £25 each in June and December to compensate them for their work with the dispensary. Reports furnished by the medical officers to the committee were read and passed at their meetings. From these medical reports it appears that during last year, when Dr Lawson held the appointment in the Under-hill District, he attended 133 cases and in course of attendance upon these cases paid 1,610 visits. At the same time the appointment in the Top-hill District was held by Dr Henley: in this district during the year, 84 cases were attended and 403 visits paid.

The secretary wrote:

> How valuable a work is done by the dispensary and how great a need is thus supplied is shewn by the eagerness with which the tickets are sought and always used up. Be it remembered the working man, as a rule, has to battle with small means all through life. Should he have a household as is not infrequently the case, like a small flock of sheep, there are many mouths to feed, many little feet to be shod, much clothes wanted; and when the rent has been paid, the wages are soon gone in providing these necessaries of life for the family. Then perhaps sickness comes, and hard times through failure of work or from some other cause, and a long doctor's bill would be a crushing climax to the poor man's troubles. It is here that the Portland Royal Dispensary comes to his aid, and proves to him the truth of the old adage that 'A friend in need is a friend indeed'.

In 1902 it was stated that 'recently the men have ceased to be recipients of the dispensary bounty owing to the action of rule 3 which states that "a family in which the united wages amount to 25 shillings a week is not to receive relief"'. In 1904, 222 cases were treated and 1,624 visits made.

The Exeter Dispensary

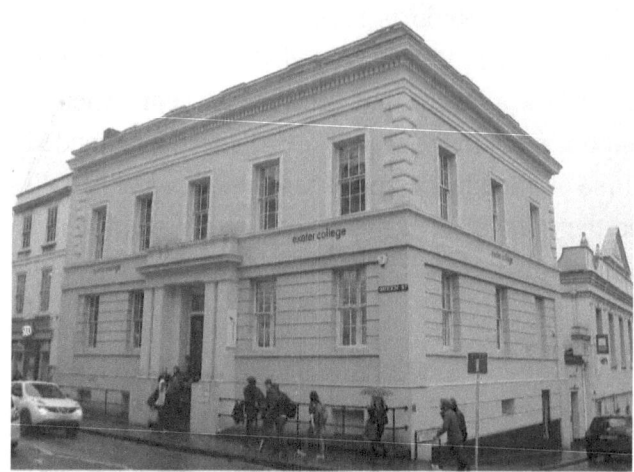

The Exeter Dispensary (now part of Exeter College); 2015.

The Exeter Dispensary was founded in 1818 by Dr Henry Blackall to provide relief for the poor suffering from fevers and contagious diseases and for children who were unfit to be admitted by the Devon and Exeter Hospital. The premises were rented for £31 per annum on Frienhay Street, and it opened for business in March. Six physicians, six surgeons, and three consultant surgeons offered their services. It was funded by subscription, with a guinea making the donor a governor of the institution. One physician and one surgeon manned the dispensary each day except Sundays, twelve doctors being appointed to do this without payment, and there were also three consultant surgeons. The work was done with no resident doctor.

Many infectious cases that would not be admitted to the Devon and Exeter Hospital were dealt with in the first nine months of operation. Whooping cough, smallpox, dysentery, scarlatina and general coughs and stomach complaints were treated. Patients were admitted at noon each day, or visited in their homes. In 1828, 9,665 cases were dealt with, and its physicians attended many of the cholera cases in the 1832 epidemic. Dr Hennis, who was killed in a duel in 1833, working from the dispensary, laboured tirelessly during the outbreak. Dr Shapter, who chronicled the epidemic in 1848, inaugurated the Devon and Exeter Pathological Society at the dispensary in the same year.

After several years of searching for a site to build a purpose designed dispensary, land on the corner of Northernhay Street and Queen Street, opposite the city prison, now the Rougemont Hotel, was acquired from the city council. The foundation stone was laid on 12 August 1840. On that day the cathedral bells were rung for what was thought to be a 'most useful charity'. Members of the governors, subscribers, and other worthies met at Congdon's subscription rooms (the Royal Subscription Rooms) and walked in procession to the cathedral for a service. After the service they then walked, accompanied by a band, to the site for the new building. The Portland stone was raised into position, and then a silver trowel was handed to Sir John Buller, who proceeded to spread a quantity of mortar, burying inside a half crown, shilling, and a sixpence. After all the usual speeches, there was a royal salute fired by General Mortimer's Fort Barbican Battery, brought from Plymouth for the occasion. They all then retired to dine at the Globe Hotel. The building, designed by Mr S A Greig, was opened in 1843 and cost £2,300.

In 1905 there were problems in the dispensary.[160] For some time the honorary medical staff and the committee had not been working together harmoniously. The first comment from the medical committee to the dispensary committee (on which there was no medical man) was that they would like their names printed in the annual report in the same manner as the lists of physicians and surgeons in the report of the Royal Devon and Exeter Hospital. Second, that the qualifications of the medical men should not be printed after their names and third that an x-ray apparatus should be provided.[161]

Later in the year at two successive meetings of the committee within one month, two gallons of brandy and two of sherry had to be authorised on each occasion, so an investigation of the use of alcohol in the dispensary was undertaken.

Table 21   Details of Alcoholic Liquors consumed at Sixteen Dispensaries

Name of Institution	Number of patients per annum	Expenditure per annum wines and brandy
Barnstaple	2831 many chronic and consumptives	Practically nil
Exeter	5400	£53
Bath Eastern	4094	About 1 pint brandy
Birmingham	54543 numerous consumptives	£5 per annum. No wine
Brighton, Hove and Preston	10,000 many chronics and consumptives	Nil
Bristol Dispensary	10556	£5 no wine
Canterbury	1672	None
Clifton	3695 200 chronics, few consumptives	6/6 (Brandy)
Dudley	4762 many chronics including 237 consumptives	Nil
Leeds	30000	£3. 3. 0
Lincoln General	3756 mostly chronics	£11. 10.0
Nottingham	14,000	Nil
Norwich	6,000 mostly acute	Nil
Plymouth Dispensary	3880	£8. 6. 0
Reading	18,000 provident members and 549 free patients	None
Worcester	1413	None
York	9215	None

The committee concluded that the consumption of alcohol in the institution seemed far in excess of that used in other dispensaries, so the attention of the medical officers was called to the matter.

The need for the x-ray equipment was rejected by the committee because the doctors wanted their private patients to use the equipment (for a fee), and the committee felt this was likely to be illegal. The medical staff were then confronted with a lengthy statement which mentioned, among other things, that the average time each medical officer devoted to each patient was one and a half minutes. Exception was taken to the time patients were kept waiting and on one occasion a medical officer was one and a half hours late and this was said to be 'generally the case'. It appeared that sometimes up to a hundred patients were waiting to see the doctors in an overcrowded and unhygienic waiting room. It was further stated that patients were decreasing. In conclusion, it was added that the only effectual remedy was the provision of a salaried medical officer whose duties would be to assist the honorary staff.

This resulted in all the honorary medical staff (eleven doctors) threatening to resign, and the committee called for a full meeting of the subscribers to deal with the matter. It was resolved within a month, and the dispensary work continued much as before.

The York Dispensary

York Dispensary was opened in 1788. At the time of its opening there were already two medical charities in York: the York County Hospital, which had been opened in 1740 as a medical and surgical hospital, and York Lunatic Asylum, opened in 1777. All three of these separate charities were supported by the subscriptions of the wealthy and treated the poor either for free or, in the case of the lunatic asylum, for modest fees.[162]

The York Dispensary, unlike York County Hospital and York Lunatic Asylum, was founded to serve the poor of York City rather than those of the County of Yorkshire. It was designed to complement the medical and surgical services offered by the County Hospital by treating the poor of the city who were suffering from chronic illnesses or other ailments which were excluded from the remit of the hospital: smallpox, measles, whooping cough, putrid sore throats, dysenteries, and all kinds of malignant fevers.

The York Dispensary was at first situated in the York Merchant Adventurers Hall, in two rooms hired for 5 guineas per annum. It saw nine hundred patients in its first year of operation and was an instant success.

In 1806 a house in St Andrewgate was purchased to provide a larger dispensary building, and, as patient numbers continued to grow, a site was purchased in New Street in 1827, to build a new, purpose designed dispensary. This opened in 1829, and the dispensary remained at New Street for the following seventy years.

Between the 1830s and '50s, the dispensary treated 2,000 to 2,500 patients each year. The local population grew, but York was in economic decline until the end of the nineteenth century, so the dispensary did useful work treating the effects of poverty on health. In the early 1880s, the dispensary saw around 4,500 to 5,000 patients each year and was again in need of expansion. By that date, the York County Hospital had also developed an extensive outpatient service used by large numbers of people; but the home visiting service offered by the dispensary remained important. In the late nineteenth century, the dispensary expanded both the boundaries it served (the city limits had expanded), and the number of full time resident medical officers it employed. From the 1880s a dental service was offered.

In 1895 the dispensary began a domiciliary maternity service, and it treated between 100 and 120 domiciliary maternity cases each year during its first few years of operation. In 1908 it was decided to additionally open a small maternity hospital. This would be for complex cases and those women with difficult home circumstances, but the main driver for its opening was that it would be a place for training pupil midwives. The maternity hospital was at 15 Ogleforth in premises initially rented and later purchased; 16 Ogleforth was also rented subsequently to increase the maternity accommodation. The maternity hospital was extremely small and treated only between 50 and 70 cases each year. At this period, York Corporation was greatly expanding its maternity and child welfare schemes, aided by government grants, in an effort to lower infant mortality. As a result, in 1922, the maternity hospital was transferred to much larger premises, in the former Acomb Hall, to the southwest of the city. This had about 40 beds and its own grounds; the domiciliary maternity service was also based there. The hospital was run jointly by the dispensary and York Corporation, but the corporation bore all running costs and soon took over the whole of the maternity service. The expense of running a maternity hospital and service had been a great drain on dispensary funds, and the maternity function was shed with considerable relief.

The numbers of persons being treated by the dispensary continued to rise, so in the 1890s the charity looked to enlarge its premises once again. A new purpose-built building in Duncombe Place was opened in 1899, with greatly extended facilities for examination and treatment. The dispensary increasingly began to take on the character of a health centre. Between seven thousand and nine thousand patients seen per year in the 1890s. Around 10 per cent of York's population attended the dispensary annually in the early 1900s.

The 1911 Insurance Act drastically affected the dispensary's patient base, as insured working people gained, under the act, free access to GPs. By 1915 dispensary patient totals had fallen by a third, to just less than five thousand per annum. But the dispensary still fulfilled a vital role in treating uninsured women, children, and the elderly, who all came to the dispensary in increasing numbers.

Financially, the interwar years were difficult ones. Like all charities with the old ticket of recommendation system, it found the system inefficient and increasingly difficult to attract a sufficient number of well-to-do subscribers. Workmen's clubs and organisations now increasingly made up the shortfall, and there were regular appeals for funding. The dispensary was no longer a prestigious place for a junior doctor to gain experience and resident medical officers were hard to recruit. Dispensary RMOs now tended to be women, and in the 1930s and '40s, many were refugees from Europe.

Despite the difficulties, the dispensary was keen to keep up to date. Clinics were extended and the dispensary began to offer increasingly specialised clinical outpatient care. In the later 1930s a programme of modernisation was begun, to provide more treatment rooms and a small operating theatre. It was probably during this modernisation process that the names on the dispensary's old nineteenth-century donation boards were recorded before the wooden boards themselves were taken down from the wall and disposed of to a local boatyard! The new facilities were completed just in time for the 150th anniversary in 1938.

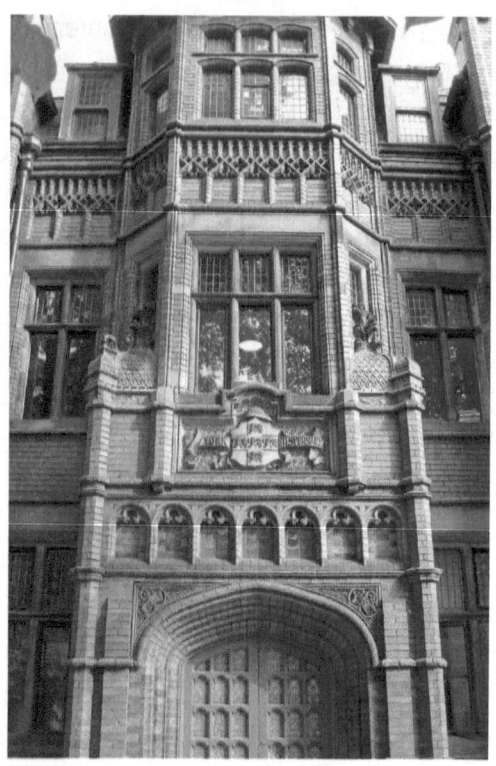

York Medical Dispensary 1898 by Edmund Kirby
of Liverpool, courtesy Sarah Cocke 2011

Newcastle-upon-Tyne Dispensary[163]

The Newcastle Dispensary started in April 1777, with those involved making it clear that the institution was not to be in opposition to the work carried out at the Infirmary and would only treat those conditions which could not be admitted there such as infectious diseases. Each subscriber of one guinea was entitled to recommend four patients per year to whom they would give a signed and printed letter of recommendation which would be presented to the resident apothecary, who noted the medicines dispensed to the patients and method by which they were to be administered. One subscription of two guineas, or a benefaction of ten guineas at one payment enabled the subscriber to become a governor and he or she could recommend eight patients per year. Those who gave larger sums could recommend a proportionate number of patients.

When the dispensary first began to operate, there were three resident physicians: Doctors Clark, Hall, and Pemberton. In the 1770s the only salaried member of the dispensary's staff was the resident apothecary, Mr William Stuart. It was the role of the apothecary to 'keep a register of the names, ages, addresses, and diseases of the patients' as well as the name of their attending physician. Originally, he was not permitted to practice outside the dispensary, but this changed as patient demand increased. Initially, the physicians and governors agreed that

> the town would be divided into seven districts; and one allotted to each physician who will visit the home patients at their own dwellings as often as circumstances of their cases shall require; and when he is prevented from attending he will procure one of his colleagues. Two physicians were to attend every Monday and Wednesday mornings with three on Friday to give advice to outpatients. Thus each physician had one outpatient session each week. Later the rota was changed to two physicians on Friday and one on Saturday.

Once in receipt of a recommendation, patients who were unable to attend the dispensary for care were instructed to send their letter to the dispensary by nine o'clock on the same day to receive a visit. Those able to attend the dispensary were to turn up before ten o'clock in the morning, where they could receive advice from one of the physicians and thereafter to attend that same physician once a week. Once a patient's course of treatment had ceased, 'they were given a ticket to return thanks the next Sunday at their parish church'. As the population of the city grew, so too did the number of patients who were treated by this institution.

In 1790 the dispensary moved to larger premises. This building consisted of a hall for the meetings of the governors, a shop and waiting room for patients, two consulting rooms for the physicians and surgeons, an electrical room, and lodgings for the apothecary and his assistant, with a small laboratory behind the building.

During the first ten years of its work, the average number of patients treated *per week* was 57. By 1800 this had increased significantly to a weekly average of 196. The number of patients treated between 1800 and 1830 remained relatively stable. Between the third and fourth decades of the nineteenth century the number of patients coming to the dispensary increased greatly to an average of more than 900 per week.

Patient demand seems to have led to a change in the admissions policy. In 1790 the committee that ran the dispensary agreed that as well as treating those patients who were in receipt of a recommendation, casual patients would also be admitted gratis. Of more than 10,000 casual patients who were admitted between 1837 and 1838, 5,331 were given just medicines; 2,002 patients required wounds to be dressed; 2,892 required some form of dental treatment (for example, had 'teeth drawn'); 358 patients were 'bleeding'; and 207 patients were admitted with burns.

Butler's study is particularly important because he describes in considerable detail the illnesses seen by the dispensary's doctors, and especially because he describes some episodes of illness as seen from the patients' and the doctor's points of view. He describes one family's illnesses as follows[164]:

> On 12 January 1779, Mary Hunter, a 13-year old girl in Newcastle, received a letter of recommendation to the dispensary, She had been confined to her bed for eight days from a continued fever. Her pulse was very fast and her teeth were black; her eyes were dull ... and she had a tickling cough. On the ninth day of her condition she was exceedingly deaf [and] very delirious.

Hunter was visited by Dr John Clark, who made detailed notes of her illness. What is interesting about Hunter is that she was not the only member of her family to have been treated by the dispensary. She was, however, the only member who received a recommendation. Mary was ill for twenty-seven days and was frequently visited by Clark until she made what appeared to have been a full recovery and 'was able to go abroad'.

Whilst Clark had been attending to Mary, her 10-year-old brother John had been 'seized with the same fever on the fifteenth day of January 1779'. John was also treated in the same way as Mary and had been prescribed with 'the bark very liberally from the beginning; and on the fifteenth day he was sensible and free from fever. Having given over his medicine, in two days he relapsed; the bark was again prescribed; and in five days more the fever totally disappeared'.

While Mary and John had both fallen ill during January, the youngest member of the family – Thomas Hunter, aged 7 years, had also been 'seized with the same fever on the second day of February'. Thomas's condition was more fragile: 'on the fourth day he passed two long worms of the *teres* kind; his fever, however, continued without the least abatement'.

Clark prescribed: twelve grains of mercury ... at bedtime. On the sixth day he had two stools, which, however, discharged no worms. For the two days following, no material alteration could be perceived. On the ninth day he vomited a long worm of the *teres* kind, and several petechial were observed upon his arms and sides. The bark was continued, and the mercurial powder was ordered to be repeated at bedtime. Clark visited Thomas until the fifteenth day of his condition, where he 'found him completely free from fever'.

The case study is important because it suggest that one single recommendation did not necessarily mean one single patient. Clearly, in a time when the homes of the poor were densely inhabited and 'fevers' prevalent, it was possible for the dispensary medical services to be more flexible than some historians previously thought.

In the next century another family experienced the following difficulties [165].

In 1839 John Groke's wife, Ellen, appealed to the mayor to get her husband into the Infirmary, and she also 'got a dispensary letter for the infant'. The family received medicines from the dispensary and were attended to by Mr Humble, one of the visiting surgeons. After two or three days in Pothouse Entry, Catherine's condition worsened. Mr Wilson of the parish tried unsuccessfully to get the three girls into All Saint's parish workhouse but was prevented by the nature of Bridget's infectious condition. Bridget's older sister Ellen was eventually sent into the workhouse, suffering from a mild cough. Mr Humble of the dispensary frequently visited Catherine and Bridget at their temporary lodgings in Sandgate.

On one of his later visits he noted that, 'I was there twice a day; in the morning the husband (John) was always groaning in bed, and in the evening he was always sitting up ... Catherine was getting worse ... I said she ought to have a little wine and water and told the mother to give it to the child ... she replied that it was of no use and that she would not torture her anymore'.

Humble gave the mixture to the child himself against her mother's protests. On the following Sunday he ordered that she (Ellen) should come to the dispensary for a blister for the child, but once again she refused. Humble attempted to reassure Catherine's mother that he 'would do all he could to save the child's life'.

Unfortunately, in reality there was little Humble could do, and the next day Catherine died from consumption. Groke's youngest daughter, Bridget, who had been the first member of the family to fall ill upon arrival in the city, was getting worse, and she died from whooping cough the following day.

Fortunately, most of the dispensary patients recovered, as is shown in the following table.

Table 22 Reported outcome of the 'recommended patients' admitted to the Newcastle Dispensary, 1780–1851:

Reported outcome	No of cases	Percentage
Cured	122,135	87.9
Relieved	1,274	0.9
Sent to Infirmary	59	0.04
Sent to fever house	97	0.06
Irregular	1,336	0.96
Refused further treatment	12	0.01
Advised to the 'country'	13	0.01
Incurable	51	0.03
Disease too advanced	50	0.03
Died	8,805	6.34
Total	138,832	100

The conditions which were commonly treated included ailments such as catarrh (possibly influenza), stomach complaints, and fevers. It is also demonstrably the case that rheumatism made up a significant proportion of admitted cases. This is not that surprising given that this condition was normally associated with heavy labour and industry and was often known by contemporaries as the coachman's disease frequently associated with muscular and joint pain. There were also considerable numbers of skin eruptions and venereal diseases treated at the dispensary. Indeed, the figures for venereal disease are probably an underestimate its presence among the poor in the city as the social stigma attached to the condition normally prohibited sufferers from appealing to a subscriber or to a hospital for care. Another interesting fact is that the number of venereal cases peak more or less during periods of warfare, when there may have been a large number soldiers and sailors in the city. Some of the other complaints recorded by the dispensary may have been related to venereal disease – for example, ulcers, skin disorders, skin eruptions, scorbutic eruptions, sore limbs, and lameness may all have been, in reality, the 'foul disease'. Retrospective diagnosis cannot, of course, be certain.

Loudon has already demonstrated that dispensaries in other port cities also commonly treated venereal cases. He found that out of more than 1,300 patients treated at the Westminster dispensary between 1775 and 1776, nearly 5 per cent suffered from venereal disease. Likewise, at the Liverpool Dispensary, between 1800 and 1801, nearly 4 per cent of all of the patients treated there laboured under this malady, these latter figures would have almost certainly been a minimum, given that as in Newcastle, the Liverpool Dispensary also treated large numbers of patients suffering from skin eruptions. However, the rules of the Bristol Dispensary in 1801 specifically stated that patients with venereal disease should not be treated.

Large numbers of children were being recommended to the dispensary, so much so that the institution appears to have been providing the most significant level of paediatric care to the poor than any other institution in Newcastle. The diseases which caused most deaths were the more dangerous conditions such as consumption, dropsy, and smallpox.

Chapter 7

DISPENSARIES IN OTHER COUNTRIES

Scotland

Andrew Duncan was appointed to teach medicine in Edinburgh in 1774 but failed to be appointed professor in 1776, so he started giving extramural lectures illustrated by using patients with chronic illnesses who were otherwise too poor to afford medical attention. In that year Duncan proposed a dispensary to provide both charitable care for the sick poor and a new additional setting in which Edinburgh's medical students could be trained. In 1777 he built a house in Surgeon's Square, near the Infirmary but the College of Surgeons prohibited the sick poor from attending Duncan's new medical academy.[166] The Royal College of Physicians of Edinburgh eventually gave him temporary accommodation for his dispensary, when he was permitted to use part of the new Physicians' Hall on George Street.

By 1783 he had sufficient funding to open the Public Dispensary on Richmond Street.

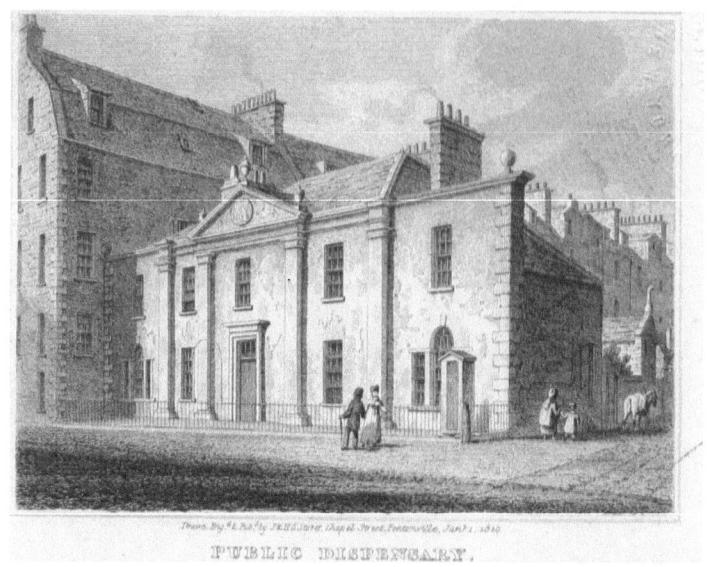

Royal Public Dispensary of Edinburgh

This was the first dispensary in Scotland and was probably modelled on the General Dispensary in Aldersgate Street in London. Patients were required to provide a letter of commendation from a subscriber or 'minister or elder of the parish in which he or she resides' confirming that 'the individual is unable to pay for medicine and is a proper object to receive medicine ... gratis'. The 'two managers ex-officio' were the presidents of the Royal College of Physicians and of the Royal College of Surgeons in Edinburgh. The tie to the colleges was strong, with all medical officers being expected to be fellows of one or either body.[167]

The workload was considerable – see table:

Table 23 Annual average patient cases Edinburgh Royal Public Dispensary

Average	General visited	Midwifery visited	Avg total visited	Dispensary patients	vaccinations	Avg total patients
1870s	1720	250	1973	6646	Approx 2000	10954
1880s	1802	170	1963	6438	Approx 500	8653

| 1890s | 2216 | 165 | 2200 | 5794 | Approx 500 | 9233 |
| 1900s | 2509 | 110 | 1620 | 5300 | | 7937 |

Source: annual report data as published in *The Scotsman*

At the Public Dispensary, Duncan also began to teach about prescribing and edited the second edition of the Edinburgh Dispensatory – a forerunner of the British National Pharmacopoeia. Medical, and subsequently pharmaceutical students studied in the dispensary's laboratory, and by 1880 the Dispensary School of Pharmacy had been developed.

In 1815 the New Town Dispensary of Edinburgh was established, which introduced midwifery practice and the visiting of patients in their homes. The Royal Dispensary soon followed suit, and medical students were able to extend their experience in the community through 'outdoor' cases.

Subsequently, the Provident Dispensary and the Livingstone Memorial Dispensary were also established in Edinburgh. According to Sutton,[168] it was not a traditional provident dispensary that encouraged prospective patients to make provision for prospective sickness in advance; the label 'provident' was used to signify a commitment to the efficacy of promoting self-sufficiency amongst the labouring classes and simply required patients to pay penny fees for medicines.

The Lancet wrote in 1898[169] that the Royal Dispensary and the so-called provident dispensary competed with each other. The average cost per patient at the Royal Dispensary was 1 shilling and one and a half pence, and the number of patients treated in the previous year was 7,224. The income was £555, of which £207 was from pupils' fees. The services of the doctors were gratuitous apart from an honorarium of £21. The number of patients was diminishing – and it was supposed that this was from the rivalry of the provident dispensary. *The Lancet* stated that the provident dispensary was lauded by its contemporaries as the most creditable illustration of a growing attempt to make the patient pay for their mercies. The total income of the institution with 9,957 patients is £219 1s 7d, of which the large sum of £100 16s and 1d consists of fees paid for prescriptions. The public, the medical officers, and the patients are all misled by such a system, which treats patients at the rate of five and a half pence a head, and, on the strength of a payment of twopence flatters them with the notion that they are paying for what they get.

The importance of undergraduate experience in dispensary practice was recognised by the medical faculty, and from 1890 onwards compulsory attendance at one of the dispensary practices became part of the Edinburgh medical curriculum. Students learned, by precept and example, the application of medicine to the individual, to the family and to the community. Cope[170] wrote 'in Scotland, the dispensary's education function and dispensary work became part of the normal curriculum of the medical student'. The senior students were organised under supervision to visit and treat the poor at home and this was a strategic response to the challenge of how to get medical students out of the lecture room.

Taking one sample year at random, from among the 198 students graduating with a normal degree at Edinburgh University in 1896, 90 per cent of the 179 students for which details are recorded had undertaken their six month training at one of the city's seven dispensaries[171] (see table).

Table 24   Total medical students attending dispensaries in 1896.

Recorded site of outpatient training	No. of students	Per cent
Royal Public Dispensary (ERPD) RPD	45	22.7
Western Dispensary	43	21.7
Edinburgh Provident Dispensary	30	15.2
EMMS Cowgate Dispensary	22	11.1
New Town Dispensary	16	8.1
At General Practitioners	9	4.5
ERPD & Royal Infirmary outpatients	2	1
Dispensary Women & Children Grove St	1	0.5
ERPD & St Anne's Dispensary	1	0.5
Western Dispensary & Royal Infirmary	1	0.5

Outside Edinburgh	9	4.5
Unspecified/unclear	19	9.6

In Glasgow there were many outdoor charities and institutions by the end of the nineteenth century, but the pattern of their development was very different from those in Edinburgh. In December 1883 a medically qualified Glasgow MP, Charles Cameron, said,[172] 'In Edinburgh, a system of dispensaries had long prevailed, in connection with which there was a staff of physicians and students, who visited the sick poor when requested, in their own homes. ... Now he had often advocated the adoption of a similar system in Glasgow without any success.'

Glasgow's two main public dispensaries of the Edinburgh type were the Glasgow Public Dispensary and Anderson's College Dispensary: both were established in the late 1870s. Anderson's closed in 1888, with Glasgow Central found in its place in 1889. Glasgow Polyklinik, established in 1885 to provide clinical material for training purposes for the Glasgow Western Medical School, provided an additional general dispensary service, although it was short-lived. Treating a reported two thousand cases per annum at the end of the 1880s, the Polyklinik offered free advice to patients but not free medicines. The Polyklinik had six speciality departments, but there is no evidence that it ever conducted home visits.[173]

The Glasgow Public Dispensary was established in 1876 to offer free advice to 'persons in necessitous circumstances, not receiving parochial relief'. It treated about twelve hundred patients a year, and patients were expected to contribute what they could towards the cost of medicines. By 1909 patients were contributing on average about a shilling a head towards the cost of treatment. The only evidence that home visiting occurred was at the Anderson's College Dispensary where it was stated: 'As with dispensaries in Edinburgh, its domiciliary work was purposefully constructed to offer senior students in their final year of study the opportunity to enhance their medical training'.

One of the physicians to the Aberdeen Dispensary at the end of the eighteenth century was Alexander Gordon. He is remembered for his publication on puerperal fever published in 1795,[174] in which he recorded the following: 'The midwife, who delivered [case number] No 3, carried the infection to No 4; from No 24 to No 25, 26, and, successively, to every woman whom she delivered'.

He continued, implicating himself in the transmission, stating: 'It is a disagreeable declaration for me to mention that I myself was the means of carrying the infection to a great number of women'.

Ireland

A few dispensaries were founded in the late eighteenth century by members of the gentry as purely private charities, but by an act of 1805 'the grand juries and the governors of county infirmaries were jointly empowered to establish dispensaries in places too distant from the infirmaries to allow the poor of those districts the advantages of convenient medical aid'.[175] Dispensary funding was entirely local and the local committee was responsible for selecting the medical officer, monitoring expenditure, establishing rules and regulations, defining the geographical extent of the dispensary district and distributing tickets to worthy recipients of the dispensary services.

The Dispensary Act was amended in 1818 in order to separate the dispensary corporations from those of the infirmaries. Their financial position was further improved by a statute of 1836 requiring, rather than permitting, grand juries to provide them with sums equal to their subscriptions. It was therefore not surprising that the numbers of dispensaries proliferated rapidly in the 1830's and by 1841 there were 615 in the country as a whole, treating in excess of 1.3 million patients.

Two factors contributed to this expansion; the subsidies from the county rates and the fact that many subscribers made their contributions conditional upon the dispensary medical officer providing free medical care for them and their families. The distribution of dispensary tickets was abused and even shopkeepers distributed tickets to customers to encourage trade. dispensary medical officers complained endlessly of such manipulation of the system by the middle and upper classes, but with little effect until 1851, when the Medical Charities Act placed the system under the supervision of the Irish Poor Law Commission.

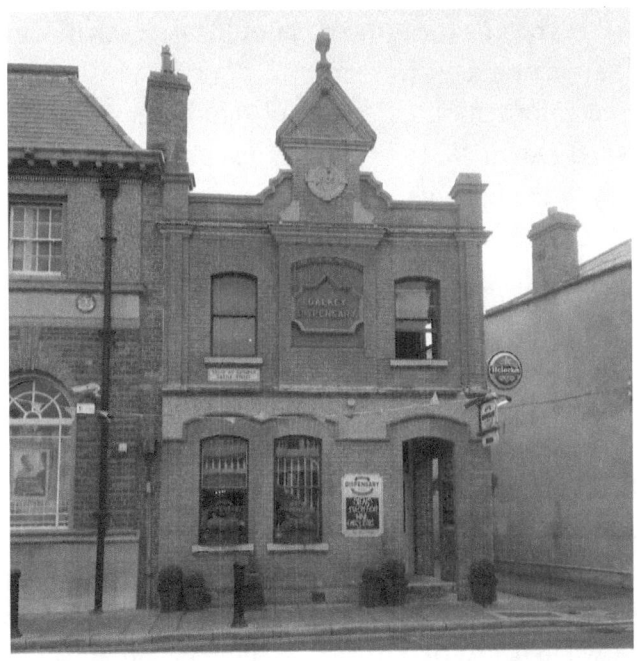

Dalkey Dispensary, Dublin. Courtesy Chris John Beckett

The dispensaries varied greatly in size and quality. Some were lavishly funded, efficient, large-scale, urban facilities, staffed by the cream of the Irish medical profession, while other were pathetic little country hovels tended by apothecaries or even medical officers with no proper credentials at all. Many appear to have been simple but adequate buildings containing rooms for the medical officer, storage facilities for the medicines, and a waiting room for patients.[176] Dispensaries were usually erected at or near workhouses.

Under the Medical Charities Act (also called the Dispensary Act) all medical officers had to have both a medical and surgical qualification. They had to be present at the dispensary during the days and hours specified by the committee. They were also to visit promptly all patients who submitted visiting tickets. Everyone requesting vaccination was offered it. No tickets were required for this. The medical officers were also required to examine and certify dangerous lunatics and were obliged for the first time to keep medical records and to furnish the committee with monthly reports. It was estimated that keeping these records would take each medical officer about half an hour a day.[177]

Detailed information exists about the dispensaries in counties Armargh and Down 1831–4.[178] It was usual for all poor persons to have access to the benefits of dispensary relief and applicants were issued with a ticket supplied and signed by a subscriber. There were two kinds of tickets: those for advice and those which entitled the bearer to receive a visit from the medical officer. The number of tickets issued to each subscriber varied widely from dispensary to dispensary. In most districts the sick were seen at the dispensary on fixed days – most were open on two or three days a week.

By 1872 there were 719 dispensary districts, 1,071 dispensaries, 801 medical officers, and 187 midwives employed in the dispensaries. In the first year of operation the dispensaries treated 690,000 persons, or approximately 11 per cent of the population, and increased that by 1863–4 when nearly 16 per cent of the population were patients.

The Irish doctors, however were not happy with dispensaries. First, they were not happy with their pay. In the mid-1850s salaries averaged less than £80 annually. The doctors felt that they should be at least £100 and more in rural districts where there was much visiting over a large area. The second irritation was over the power of the Poor Law Commission. If a doctor was accused of some charge, the investigation took place *in camera* and was without appeal. Finally, the doctors were increasingly disturbed by the rampant abuse of dispensary ticket distribution by committee members. Throughout the nineteenth century Irish physicians and surgeons insisted on the traditional guinea fee from their private patients – it was apparently seen as indicating the profession's sense of dignity. In 1868 the average wage in Ireland amounted to 7 shillings a week, making three times this an almost impossible sum for the poor and middle classes to pay – hence needing to access dispensary care.

The United States of America

As in the United Kingdom, the first dispensaries were founded in the late eighteenth century in Philadelphia (1786), New York (1791), Boston (1796), and Baltimore (1800); they also started with subscribers and the issuing of tickets to the poor. They grew slowly in number through the mid-nineteenth century and remained concentrated in the East.[179] By 1874 there were twenty-nine dispensaries in New York and by 1877, thirty-three in Philadelphia. Operating on small budgets, their main resource was the free service of part-time physicians, who used them to teach medical students, gain experience in diagnosis and advance their careers. The more medical students in need of opportunities for training, the more dispensaries were established.

Almost all dispensaries had a central building, with the prominent exception of Boston, which had none until the 1850s, and usually employed one full-time apothecary or house physician who acted as steward, performed minor surgery, often vaccinated, and pulled teeth, as well as prescribing for some patients.[180] Most of the dispensaries existed with very limited budgets as indicated by how often they had to rent out parts of the dispensary premises to commercial tenants.[181] An example of the pressure management put on the doctors on occasions when there was little money was when in 1844, the Boston Dispensary managers sought to compel their visiting physicians to employ scarification and bleeding rather than the far more expensive leeches.[182] The physicians argued not only that the leeches had a different physiological effect but that they had well-nigh banished more painful modes of bloodletting from private practice. As medical schools increased in number during the late nineteenth century, dispensaries did too. By 1900 there were an estimated one hundred in the country, and by 1916 there were 680.[183]

The rules of the Baltimore Dispensary[184] in 1803 stated that each subscriber paid $5 a year or $50 as a single payment. That there would be a board of twelve managers elected by the donors to regulate the affairs of the institution and they should meet monthly. Three attending physicians were to be appointed annually who would make a report to the managers about the patients they had seen and what diseases they had treated and whether in the dispensary or at the patients' homes. These physicians received salaries according to their workload. Four consulting physicians were also appointed and the attending physicians could consult them over difficult or complicated cases. There was one apothecary who lived in the dispensary and he had to devote his whole time to the work. The dispensary was open from 8 a.m. until 2 p.m. and from 3 p.m. until sunset on every day except Sunday, when the dispensary was closed from 11 a.m. to 5 p.m. The physicians attended for one hour each day and then did visits. There were 1,067 patients in the year.

There was considerable criticism of the growth of the dispensaries as many doctors claimed that that patients who used them could well pay for their medical services. This 'dispensary abuse' was, according to Starr,[185] in large measure a conflict between two segments of the medical profession; the economically insecure general practitioners who saw the dispensaries as depriving them of income; and the more privileged specialists, or would-be specialists, who used the dispensary for teaching, research, and the acquisition of professional connections. The former wanted charity limited and the private market kept as large as possible. The latter wanted no limit on their prerogative to accept 'interesting' cases, even if that meant occasionally taking patients who might be able to afford private treatment.

The emphasis placed on medical specialities that has characterised medical practice in the United States over the last century can be recognised as early as 1826 when the New York dispensary reorganised itself, dividing patients into 'classes' according to the nature of their ailment. By mid-century the need for speciality differentiation was unquestioned. When the Brooklyn Dispensary opened in 1847, for example, it announced that patients would be distributed among the following classes: women and children, heart, lungs and throat, skin and vaccination, head and digestive organs, eye and ear, surgery and unclassified diseases. In the late-nineteenth century, specialized dispensaries became increasingly established.

Immigration was one of the other problems faced by the East Coast dispensaries. In 1853 the New York Dispensary's patients consisted of 1,583 born in the United States and 4,886 born in Ireland. At the Philadelphia Dispensary in 1857, 1,906 patients were born in the United States and 3,649 in Ireland. A Boston Dispensary physician complained that 'deserving American poor were often deterred from seeking aid because they shrink from seeming to place themselves on a level with the degraded classes among the Irish'. The unfamiliar attitudes and habits of these patients added to their troublesomeness; they ignored hygienic advice and often denied the physician's simplest requests.

Later, Jews and Italians replaced the Irish as objects of the dispensary physician's frustration and disdain.[186]

In 1916 it was estimated that there were 760 dispensaries in the United States,[187] of which 400 were general dispensaries, 300 were for tuberculosis only, and 60 were restricted to specialities. Apparently, there had been a sevenfold increase in the number of dispensaries since 1900 and only ten states had no dispensaries at all. Of the 400 general dispensaries, about 62.5 per cent were outpatient departments of hospitals.

The fate of the dispensaries was linked to reform of medical education as the abuses of the dispensary system stemmed from the proliferation of medical schools. After the profession was able to rid itself of many of the medical schools in the first two decades of the twentieth century, the pool of free labour for dispensaries disappeared. Dispensaries disappeared as free standing institutions; many were absorbed into hospitals as outpatient departments, which by the twenties were imposing charges on patients from whom a fee could be collected.

So dispensaries have disappeared in the United Kingdom and in the United States. As Starr[188] has written: like hospitals, dispensaries were originally established as charities for the poor, but unlike hospitals, they failed to make the transition to serving society as a whole. Had different forces shaped the system, the dispensary rather than the hospital might have become the nucleus for community medical services, but this was not the direction events took.

Rosenberg[189] concluded that the death of the dispensary and the transfer of its functions and client constituency to general hospitals has not be an unqualified success.

Australia

The Sydney Dispensary was created in 1826 to provide outpatient care for 'free poor persons, unable to pay for medical attendance'. It was conducted in traditional charitable lines and operated from several city premises before obtaining the south wing of the Rum Hospital in 1845 where it remained until 1848. It then expanded to serve inpatients and changed its name to the Sydney Infirmary and Dispensary, a title officially approved in 1844.[190]

The Sydney Dispensary had no beds and limited its operation to patients able to attend the dispensary, and the visits of the resident surgeon to patients. The numbers of patients increased in each year from 1835: 566 in 1836 to 2,057 in 1843. The countries the patients came from during September, October, November, and December 1843 were England, 146; Scotland, 38; Ireland, 400; native-born, 217; West Indies, 3; United States, 2; Canadians, 3; and one each from New Zealand, East Indies, Germany, and Sweden. There were 59 cases of abscess; 157 of constipation and dyspepsia; 200 of diarrhoea and dysentery; 330 of inflammation; 31 of whooping-cough; 142 of ulcers.

The total receipts for 1843 were £202 19s. Expenses included the salary of Dr. McKellar, £130 ; Mr. Houston (the dispenser), £75; Housekeeper, £9 15s. ; Medicine, £25 5s. 7d. ; Printing, £47 9s. 9d. [191]

In Melbourne a homoeopathic dispensary was started in 1869. It was open on Mondays, Wednesdays, and Fridays from 9 to 10 a.m. and had three honorary medical officers. During the first eleven months of its existence, 741 patients were seen. Each governor was entitled to four recommendations per guinea subscribed. It had a very chequered history and became the allopathic Prince Henry's Hospital in 1936.

India

Sir Henry C Burdett, in 1893 claimed that the 'dispensary system of India forms the most striking feature of its medical history'. Blake[192] states that the dispensary movement can be seen as a decisive factor in the history of colonial medicine in India, shaping attitudes and opinions about the level of medical care which should be provided, what kind, and for whom. It provided an inducement and a convenient site to study the effects of disease on the Indian body, raising hopes that any knowledge gained would in turn provide better protection for those Europeans unused to the heat and different disease environment.

The Edinburgh Medical Missionary Society was formed in 1841. It was not a religious organisation but its membership supplied physicians to many of the church based missionary societies to which they personally belonged Their training ground was the charitable dispensary in Cowgate, Edinburgh, and, not surprisingly, many ended up in India.

In 1809 there was one dispensary in Bombay Presidency, the Bombay Native Hospital, but in 1875 there were 118 dispensaries. The dispensaries were therefore popular, and retained their popularity throughout the century. However, there were too few for the large and scattered population and some may argue that they may not have been the most striking feature in India's medical history, but they did make an impact on the poor who gained access.

Harrison[193] states that the establishment of charitable dispensaries from the 1830s was one of the earliest attempts to provide Western medical care for the Indian people. Many of the early dispensaries in Bengal owed their existence to Indian philanthropists who provided the money for the building of dispensary houses and a monthly sum for maintenance. After 1860, funds came from commercial organisations, from Europeans, and from some government contributions.

The number of dispensaries increased considerably after 1870. In 1867 there were 61 dispensaries in Bengal, with 17,000 inpatients and 318,895 outpatients, but by 1900 more than 500 had been established in Bengal, with more than two million outpatients. A similar situation was occurring in Bombay with the number of beds in dispensaries increasing from 764 to 1883 between the years 1880 and 1908.[194]

The large number of inpatients indicate that Indian dispensaries were very different from those in other countries. Other differences include the difficulty of managing the dispensaries with many varieties of doctors.[195] I have found no evidence that subscribers had to recommend patients to the dispensaries in India.

France

There is little information about dispensaries in France, but one report[196] stated that in 1818, the Philanthropic Society of Paris has established five dispensaries, three to the south and two to the north of the Seine in the midst of the most populous districts of the city, nearly on the same footing as those in London. The admissions into these dispensaries amount to about 1,600, being rather more than one fourth of the number admitted by the Westminster General Dispensary in the course of a year.

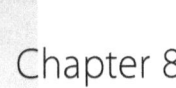

Chapter 8

THE PROVIDENT
DISPENSARIES

In 1832 John Storer, MD, FRS, consulting physician to the Nottingham Infirmary, published a book titled *Hints on the Constitution of Dispensaries*.[197] In this, he described the two main objections to the voluntary dispensaries: first that doctors spend a significant amount of time each week caring for the poor without any financial recompense, whereas the subscribers simply meet together for an hour or so once a month. Second, that many poor families, who would normally pay for medical care, now attend the dispensaries at no cost as the service is free. He supported the proposals that had been put forward by Dr Smith of Warwick and the subscribers of the Derby Dispensary where there were three classes of patients: the free subscribers who would regularly contribute a small sum each month to enable their families to attend the Dispensary at times of illness without cost; the normal charity patients; and the parish poor.

Dr AP Stewart, physician to the St Pancras Royal General Dispensary, wrote in 1850 that 'the reliance of the poor on charitable aid increases as fast as assistance is provided and outstrips the natural growth of population, so that it may be inferred that this loss in independence results in great degree from the provision made to supply the wants of in-frugal and improvident people'.[198]

Whatever we may think about this statement, there is no doubt that many in the middle of the nineteenth century were becoming concerned about the increasing reliance of many poor people on charity.

In an attempt to counter this reliance on charity, at least 39 provident dispensaries were formed in England and Wales by 1875. These were initially promoted by Dr Henry Lilley Smith,[199] who wrote about them in 1850 when he claimed that he had been developing the idea for more than thirty years. The principle was that the new form of dispensaries was supported by the beneficiaries as well as the more opulent donors.

Smith described how the Royal Victoria Dispensary at Northampton worked in the following ways:

- The funds were derived from the subscriptions and donations of honorary members, and the payments of free members.
- The honorary fund bore the expenses of the institution; the free members' fund paid for the cost of drugs and what was left over was divided among the medical officers.
- The institution was managed by a president and committee elected from the honorary members.
- The medical officers attend daily in rotation and all doctors practising in the area shall be considered unless they decline, as medical officers.
- The free members shall consist of working persons and servants, their wives and children, not receiving parish relief, and being unable to pay for medical advice in the normal way.

Every free member 14 and older had to pay a penny, and under that age a half penny a week; twopence a week was the charge for a man, wife, and all children 14 and younger. All payments had to be paid in advance and no one with an illness was admitted to the scheme unless they paid an entrance fee of five shillings.

Every free member had a choice of whichever medical officer he may prefer, but he was not allowed to change that medical attendant during the course of an illness without the permission of the committee. Married women who were free members could obtain the attendance of a medical officer at her confinement by paying five shillings, which was subsequently handed to the medical officer.

The Lancet printed the dispensary's account sheet in 1850, showing that one doctor had attended nearly 3,000 patients at the dispensary, at home, or in confinement and had received more than £130. Another attended a total of 1,400 and received £55; a third saw more than 300 and received £14; a fourth saw 200 for £13; and a fifth saw 120 for £4 16s.[200] The total remuneration of £220 had been the sum leftover after all other expenses had been paid out of the contributions. The *Lancet* concluded that as payment was less than eightpence a case, were the committee quite certain that the people attended were really poor, or were the medical officers being robbed?

Twenty years later *The Lancet* undertook an investigation. In 1870 contributions amounted to nearly £1,900, of this £400 was appropriated for drugs and other expenses and £1,500 divided amongst the three medical officers in proportion to the number of patients attended. More than 50,000 cases had been seen, of which 17,000 had been in the homes of the poor, and more than 62,000 prescriptions had been made

The provident dispensary movement was suggested as an answer to the huge numbers of poor people attending hospital outpatient departments in the middle of the nineteenth century, particularly in London. The situation in Bristol at the Infirmary outpatient department was no different and was described as follows[201]:

In 1854 the trustees decided to limit the number of outpatients that could be recommended by a subscriber of two guineas a year to six a year. There were two rooms for seeing these outpatients, one medical and one surgical, and a common room in which all, both male and female, waited their turn. Until 1860, when outpatients could be seen on every weekday, outpatients were seen on Monday and Thursday mornings only at 11 a.m., and on each of these days there were two physicians seated at a table in the medical room and two or three surgeons in the surgical room attending to their patients at the same time. The atmosphere in the room in which these patients waited was described as 'tainted and poisonous'. A policeman was employed to keep order, and when a fresh 'batch' was wanted, the door of the common room was opened by one or two attendants, and the crowd of maimed and diseased wretches shouldered and fought their way into the place where they were seen by the physicians and surgeons who had to arrange and sort them as they came in. It was not until 1859 that one of the resident officers sorted the cases into medical and surgical beforehand. Men and women were, under this old system, admitted into the room, where they were examined and attended together, and the great indelicacy of this arrangement was obvious.

Following the development of the Charity Organisation Society in 1869, Sir Charles Trevelyan showed how its principles could be applied to medical charities in general. He believed that the existing system not only failed to meet current needs but 'exercised a depressing and corrupting influence on the character of the working classes'.

To relieve pressure on hospital outpatient departments and on hospital funds, he proposed a system of provident dispensaries based on the insurance principle. He said people should be compelled to adopt habits of self-respect and industry, so that outpatient departments could be rid of medical mendicants. At an early meeting the subcommittee discussed the influence that could be applied to the government to enquire into the publication of hospital and dispensary accounts. In 1874 it proceeded to examine the advantages and disadvantages of governors' letters (or subscribers' tickets) and concluded that the system should be abolished as soon as public opinion was ready for the change.[202]

In Bristol, a number of small provident dispensaries were set up but provident dispensaries never became a major part of the medical services in that city. Apparently the Annual Report of the Bristol General Hospital in 1880 stated that the committee hoped the outpatient department of that hospital should become more and more a Provident Dispensary.[203]

'The workmen's contributions, together with the deposit for bottles, was sufficient to provide a fund of 1s. 3d. per head for all the outpatients admitted during the year; thus making this department a provident dispensary'.

Symes added,[204] 'Today [1932] the Health Insurance Act and panel practice have modified this view, and the tendency is for the outpatient department to be more and more on a consultative basis'.

The Haverstock Hill and Maldon Road Provident Dispensary in London was founded in 1865 and is a good example of how a provident dispensary was run.[205]

- There were two funds within the dispensary: the Free Members' fund formed by the monthly subscriptions of the 'free' members and the honorary fund that was supported by the affluent residents. The honorary fund paid for the working expenses, rent, furniture, coal, gas, dispenser's salary, and (rather surprisingly) quinine and cod liver oil. It also contributed to the midwifery expenses. The Free Members' fund paid the drugs bill (apart from quinine and cod liver oil), and the remainder was divided among the medical officers according to the amount of work they did. This meant, of course, that there was an incentive for the medical officers to economise on the drugs they prescribed!
- There were three medical officers, and patients could choose which doctor to consult. Each one attended the dispensary on two days a week and visited patients at home if necessary.
- An ideal patient was a man with a family earning no more than 30 shillings a week (equivalent to just less than £70 a week in 2005). People had to be admitted at least a month before they could access care, unless they were prepared to pay 5 shillings 'up front'. Adult males and married women paid sixpence a month; a man and his wife, eightpence, which

was increased in proportion to the number of children, up to one shilling and four pence.

- Midwifery costs were £1 15s from the patient to the doctor, and in addition, the doctor received 5 shillings from the honorary fund. But if the member preferred it, the midwife of the institution would attend for a small fee and could be assisted by a medical officer if there were difficulties when the patient would pay 3 shillings, and 7 shillings would be paid from the honorary fund.
- The dispensary was managed by a committee of the honorary subscribers, and the medical officers were members *ex officio*. Some other dispensaries had free members on the committee, and it was reported to work well.

During 1869, £265 was divided amongst the three medical officers. For this, fifteen visits daily, on average, were made (five by each doctor), and fifteen patients were seen in the dispensary.

Dr Anderson, one of the medical officers, wrote: 'I have found provident dispensary patients less exacting, and more grateful, and more thoughtful of their doctor than charitable dispensary patients'.

He went on to say that he believed provident dispensaries would never be able to prosper while there are charitable hospitals and dispensaries to which it is respectable for patients to turn.

In London the Metropolitan Provident Medical Association was founded in 1881 to 'relieve hospital abuse and to extend self-supporting and self-governing provident dispensaries throughout the metropolis'. It was designed to cover the whole of the city with a target of fifty branches (although there were only twenty-one in 1902). The members paid 6d a month if a single man, 10d per month if a married couple, and 2d a month for up to three children younger than 14; the remaining children were not charged for. Members had the right to choose which practitioner they saw and could also be treated in their own homes if need be; each dispensary also provided medicines, had a midwife and dentist, and sent out for trained nurses when necessary.[206]

The work of one of its dispensaries was described by Wunderlich[207]. He described the work of the Tottenham branch that had been in existence for ten years, and, in particular, his own case load at the end of the nineteenth century. He described how members joined to ensure that mothers and young children obtained care with the many minor illnesses that occur during that stage of life. He concluded that members leave the association when these needs disappear and that the purpose of the association being there is to provide medical help at times of accident or serious illness, and therefore being able to prevent the way that people use the hospitals. He found that the membership changed by 16 per cent a year and that he had not been called to treat 'cases of acute and organic disease' during the three years he worked for the branch. Most members consulted at least once during the year.

The following table shows the growth of Provident dispensaries in London. In the provinces it was even greater.

Table 25   The Provident Dispensaries in London[208]

Name	Location	Founded	Annual Income	Patients/ year	Cost/ patient
St Marylebone	6 Charlotte St	1833	394	3596	2s 2d
Poplar Medical Association	Town Hall	1836			
Paddington	104 Start St	1837	431	7261	1s 2d
Battersea*	High St, Battersea	1844			
St John's Wood & Portland Town	Henstridge Villas	1844	326	1051	6s 3d
Hampstead	New End	1845			
East London	495 Commercial Rd	1846			
Clapham General	42 Manor St	1849	461	3564	2s 6d
North Pancras	30 Hawley Cres	1850	64	225	5s 7d
Central Pancras	112 Drummond St	1853	70		
Westbourne	Bishop's Rd	1855	272	2249	2s 5d
Notting Hill*	43 Portland Rd	1860			
Camberwell	Camberwell Green	1862	1902		

Wandsworth	SW	1863		
Forest Hill	73 Perry Rd	1865		
Haverstock Hill & Malden Rd	132 Malden Rd	1865	330	3168
St George's	Little Grosvenor St	1868	407	
Childs Hill and Cricklewood		1872		
Provident Surgical Appliance Soc	12 Finsbury Circus	1872		
Western	Rochester Row	1874	1396	4456
Kilburn	1 Greville Rd	1875		
Lewisham, Ladywell &Hither Green	Ladywell	1876		
Brompton and Knightsbridge	28 Fulham Rd	1877	1910	
Hackney*	14 Brett Rd	1877		
Deptford*	437 New Cross Rd	1878		
Wandsworth Com & Upper Tooting	Bolingbroke House	1878		
Lewisham Self Supporting	29 High Street	1880		
Metropolitan Medical Association	5 Lamb's Conduit	1880		
Bloomsbury*	5 Lamb's Conduit	1881		
Clerkenwell & St Luke's Club*	George's Rd	1881		
Medical Aid Friendly Society	117 New Rd	1881		
Soho and St James' Medical Club*	Haymarket	1881		
Kensal Town	43 Golborne Rd	1881		
Croydon*	12 Katharine St	1881		
Pimlico	68 Lupus St	1882		
Camden Town*	62 Camden Road	1884		
Greenwich	24 Nelson St	1885		

East Dulwich	Landell's Rd	1886
Tottenham Medical Club*	166 High Rd	1887
Whitechapel	137 Whitechapel Rd	1889
Chelsea*	472 King's Rd	1891
Blackfriars	Blackfriars Rd	1894
Edmonton Medical Club*	161 Fore Street	1894
Woolwich, Plumstead & Charlton	6 Russell Place	1894
Islington Medical Club*	5 Thornhill Cresc	1896
Leman Street*	19 Leman St	1898

*A branch of the Metropolitan Provident Medical Association

The Warwick Provident Sick Association (WPSA)

This was established in 1857 by the Rev. Edwin Trevelyan Smith, the vicar of St Paul's in West Warwick, and originally intended for working men of that parish. Mid-century controversy about provident dispensaries erupted locally in 1858, with different outcomes for the two Warwick institutions. Dr HL Smith delivered an emotional speech at a public meeting. He advocated the establishment of a number of 'Victoria provident dispensaries' to mark the queen's visit to Warwickshire that year. The ensuing debate was heated, even rancorous, each side accusing the other of bad faith and culpable ignorance. Smith asserted that the working man gained dignity and independence by contributing to the cost of his medical care. His opponents' case was that Warwick differed from manufacturing towns in its prevalent poverty, with much casual or seasonal work and a lack of well-paid reliable employment. A strongly worded 'memorial' in January 1859, albeit signed by peers and prominent county figures, failed to move the Warwick Dispensary. Its committee remained unconvinced by Smith's arguments, and certain medical officers were vehemently opposed.

In contrast, the Provident Sick Association in June 1859 changed its rules and adopted the new name of the Warwick Provident Dispensary. It was open to working people and the families 'unable to pay for medical attendance in the usual way', but not receiving parish relief, and to domestic servants earning less than £8 annually. Their contributions were a penny a week or 2d for a man, his wife, and his children 14 and younger. The work was supported by voluntary contributions from the prosperous, while local noblemen and gentlemen were appointed president and vice presidents. Despite the name it seems there was no dedicated dispensary building, members being treated at the houses of its two surgeons. Over time nearby parishes joined the scheme, and in 1864 a branch was formed in the industrial suburb of Emscote, managed by the local vicar (the Rev HB Dickins) and a manufacturer (George Nelson). The membership steadily increased, with a total of 325 in 1867 and 382 in 1870 (181 of whom were in Warwick town).

In 1870 the Warwick Dispensary committee inquired among self-supporting institutions in the Midlands as to the practicalities of the provident system. After encouraging replies, especially as regards the ability of the poorly paid to manage weekly penny subscriptions (or 2d for a family), the committee changed its policy. Some members remained opposed, including two medical officers who resigned. The dispensary did retain the system of free tickets issued by a governor, but now for use only in cases of destitution or emergency. After two months' treatment the free ticket holder was required to become a provident member. In 1871 the two institutions amalgamated under the name of the Warwick Provident Dispensary, adopting 8 Castle Street as the base.

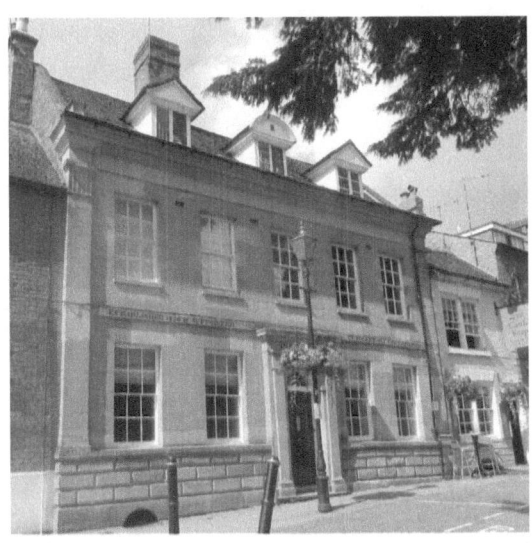

The Old Dispensary, 8 Castle Street, Warwick (now
a private house). Photo courtesy John Wilmot.

During January 1871, the first month of the new system, 530
individuals from 207 families applied to join, the number reaching
1,930 (700 families) by the year's end. By 1874 the dispensary had
3,010 provident members, and despite some fluctuations, the number
rose to 4,456 in 1911.[209]

Prospective members applied to the secretary who entered the
name, address, ages and occupation of the applicant in large ledgers,
which were presented to the committee at its weekly meetings. The
most prosperous artisans were barred at Warwick through a weekly
income limit of 30 shillings. After paying the first month's subscription
(4d for a single person and 8d for a family) members received a
booklet summarising the rules and opening hours, with space for
prescriptions to be prepared by the dispenser. The honorary secretary
was in charge of everyday administration. The dispenser collected
members' weekly payments and a collector called on subscribers
annually. By 1881 the three medical officers each attended at the
dispensary twice weekly as well as making home visits.

Each patient entered an oak-panelled waiting room furnished
with benches. They saw a doctor before taking prescriptions to be

prepared by the dispenser in the front room. The doctors were seeing one hundred new patients each week and performed the necessary midwifery with about forty cases most years. The dispensary introduced free dentistry around 1871 with about forty to fifty cases each year. A cottage hospital opened in the upstairs space in 1874. Prospective patients needed a subscriber's recommendation and paid an admission fee of 2s 6d, followed by 1s and 3d each week. In 1891 three bedrooms held five beds for patients, and a further bedroom was used by the resident matron-housekeeper.

Derby Dispensary

In 1830 Dr HL Smith gave a lecture to the Derby Medical Society on the subject of his dispensary system, but the doctors rejected by one vote a proposal to start such a dispensary in Derby. Dr John Jones was not put off, and with some local citizens, he established the Derby Self-Supporting Charitable and Parochial Dispensary.[210] In 1844, with the dispensary nearly insolvent as a result of a large reduction in the number of subscribers, it was decided to discontinue the 'charity class' of patients, and the dispensary remodelled as a provident dispensary with the aim of 'placing medical aid within the means of the working classes'.

The rules of the dispensary were as follows:

- The funds were derived from two sources: from small weekly payments of subscribers termed 'free members' and from more affluent 'honorary members' who, on payment of 10 guineas, would become life governors; or annual subscribers of one guinea became governors for that year.
- The income from subscribers formed a fund from which the expenses of the institution were paid. If there was any surplus, it was given to the surgeons according to the number of patients registered to him.

- There was a medical and a non-medical secretary, and one was present each Thursday for admitting free members and receiving their weekly contributions. The committee members met every month.

- Each free member subscribed one penny a week and had to nominate his or her medical officer. Patients could not be admitted when sick unless they paid in advance 3 shillings and sixpence for adults and one shilling and ninepence for those 14 or younger, together with their weekly contributions. Married women could be attended during their confinements by the surgeon of their choice by depositing 7 shillings before having their baby.

- A dispenser was appointed by the committee, and he lived at the dispensary and opened it every morning (except Sunday) at 9 a.m. and closed it at 8 p.m. He had to prepare prescriptions at any hour in emergencies. On Sundays the dispensary was open from 8 a.m. and closed at 10 a.m. He had to register the name and address and complaints of every patient.

- Eight surgeons and one physician were appointed by ballot at the annual meeting. The surgeons attended daily in rotation and at appointed hours, but when the patients were too ill to attend, they were visited at their homes. There was a note added to this rule saying that 'the medical officers generally disregard this rule and prefer making arrangements with the patients to see them at their own surgeries instead of at the dispensary'. The surgeons retired after three years and could seek re-election. They had to keep a register of the name, age, and address with the results and any comments.

What Was Going on in Leicester?

The Leicester General Dispensary was founded in 1833. This was supported by six surgeons and one physician who gave their services freely together with a salaried medical officer. They saw about 1,550 patients each year. A provident dispensary was formed in 1862. In 1895 the British Medical Association (BMA) described the situation in Leicester,[211] where, it was claimed, existed a successful provident dispensary. There the patient paid one penny a week. The BMA compared the principles of thrift and providence with what went on in practice and stated that the practice of these virtues brought into view many sordid motives and unpleasant details.

The journal provided details of the costs involved.[212] The artisan paid his one penny a week for medical attendance, and thinking this went to the doctor, imagined he had done his duty in providing for a rainy day. But his one penny did not go to the doctor; in fact, the doctor got 1 shilling 10.9 pence per year, less than half the adult annual subscription. The rest went to 'management'. The medical officers received £3,530; drugs cost £795; and the surgeon-dentist received £15 – a total of £4,341, or 70 per cent of the sum paid. The 30 per cent remaining included the manager's salary (£600) and the collector's wages (£396).

The critical article goes on to say that this provident system would have gone to the dogs years ago but for the charitable contributions such as subscriptions, donations, and legacies. The conclusion was that the dispensary was in no sense self-supporting but was still a charity and was constantly in debt.

Occasionally, small provident dispensaries were set up in small towns, such as Wantage, Oxfordshire, which resulted from a legacy left by Mrs Harriet Firth who bequeathed £2,000 for the establishment and maintenance of a medical dispensary for Wantage and the neighbourhood.[213] The dispensary was established in 1888 and became provident in 1893. The legacy produced an annual income of about £72, which was about a third of the dispensary's annual income – the remainder coming from patients' contributions. On payment of a nominal weekly sum, the working men and their families would receive free medical treatment at the surgeries of local doctors and home visits if they were very ill. Each provident member 14 years or older paid 1d per week and 3d for a family and all children 14 years of age or younger. Members had to show their admission ticket and attend the surgery between 9.30 and 10.30 in the morning and bring their own bottles and gallipots with them. On Sundays the surgery was only open for urgent cases at 9.30 a.m. In 1909, out of a population of 3,766, there were 131 families subscribing £159 in the year. The expenses were £20 for the bookkeeper's salary, and rent and insurance £11, and the balance (£197) was divided among the medical officers. This dispensary continued functioning until 1947.

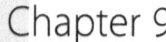

Chapter 9

CAN WE LEARN ANYTHING FROM THE DISPENSARIES?

Since history has no properly scientific value, its only purpose is educative. And if historians neglect to educate the public, if they fail to interest it intelligently in the past, then all their historical learning is valueless except in so far as it educates themselves.—GM Trevelyan

The study of history is the best medicine for a sick mind; for in history you have a record of the infinite variety of human experience plainly set out for all to see; and in that record you can find yourself and your country both examples and warnings; fine things to take as models, base things rotten through and through, to avoid. —Livy (Titus Livius)

Having seen something of the way the dispensaries provided a medical service for poor patients we can summarise the advantages and disadvantages of this system of health care. See Table 1.

Table 26 What Did the Dispensaries Offer to Patients, Doctors, and Subscribers?

	To patients	To doctors	To subscribers
Acute illnesses in the family	If low income and previously working, could request a ticket from a subscriber and obtain free medical advice either in dispensary or at home. Most offered free vaccination against small pox.	An obligation to advise and treat the presenting medical problem for free if a physician or surgeon	Were aware of the illnesses and social conditions being experienced in neighbouring families and the district
Were there restrictions?	Patient or family had to be 'deserving poor'. A ticket had to be obtained. Antenatal mother had to be married to have care during delivery. Patient had to live within limited area. Patients had to usually provide containers for medicines.	Doctors had to have suitable qualifications and were selected. Junior doctors had usually to be resident or live close by. Resident doctors were not allowed to have private patients until they had been employed for a few years.	None apart from being willing to subscribe at least 10s 6d per year or to make a substantial donation

Advantages in attending the dispensary	Guarantee of help	Became well-known to patients and subscribers and likely to get secondary financial rewards. Saw a wide range of medical problems and had the opportunity of observing the progress of illnesses. Research and teaching opportunities	Being viewed as philanthropic, especially if became involved in the various committees associated with the dispensary
Disadvantages of being associated with the dispensary	No choice of doctor Demeaning to have to obtain a ticket	Being liable to control by the committee	Having to raise sufficient money each year to run the dispensary
Advantages of provident dispensary	Patients and families insure provision of health care and can see a particular doctor	Patients are now involved and 'partners' in health care. Regular income	Less need for fundraising
Disadvantages of provident dispensary	Increasing expectations of quality of care		Need to provide staff to collect subscriptions and monitor budget carefully

Dispensaries formed a key part of medical practice for about two hundred years before the NHS was created in 1948, yet all trace of them as medical institutions has disappeared. Under the National Health Service Act of 1946, most of the country's voluntary hospitals, clinics, and dispensaries were transferred to the NHS by 1948. From the beginning of the NHS, patients were freely cared for by hospitals, general practitioners, and the public health services. Dispensaries funded by subscriptions disappeared overnight. Those institutions run by subscribers were no longer needed.

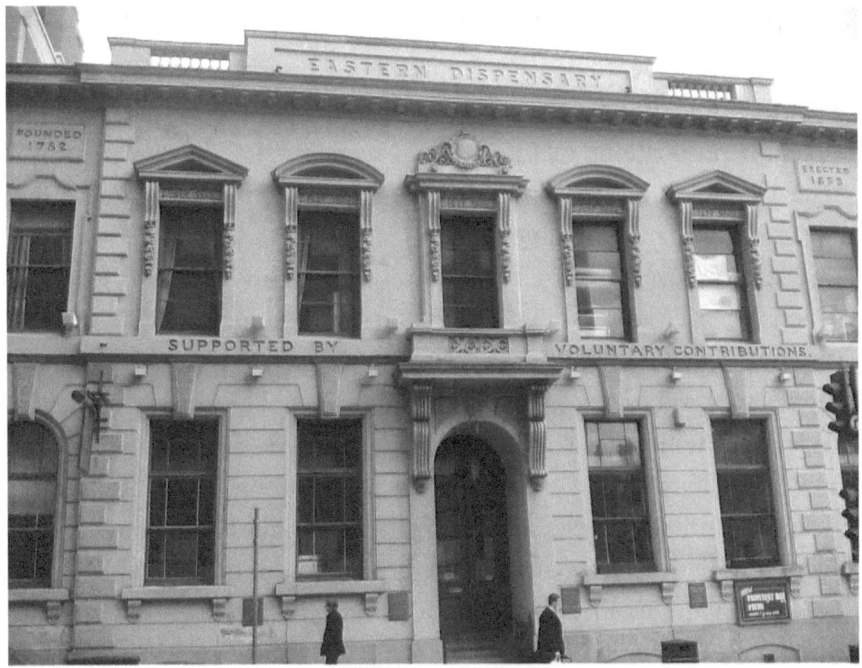

The Eastern Dispensary, Leman Street, London,
now a restaurant, courtesy Ewan Munro.

So, What Has Been Lost?

1. The Subscriber System

The subscriber system of funding institutions to look after the medical problems of the poor, where the subscriber has the right to introduce the patient to the dispensary by handing over a note is a historical oddity. It ensured that the wealthy donor developed a relationship with the poor patient, even though the relationship may not have lasted a long time. In many ways a relationship like this can be considered appropriate and will have brought many wealthy people knowledge of the problems faced by the poor; but on the other hand this sort of dependent relationship can be seen as totally inappropriate and demeaning. The notes or tickets would have been handed to the 'deserving' poor rather than paupers and beggars who would most likely have been directed to the poorhouse. Towards the end of the nineteenth century a number of the dispensaries, such as at Clifton and Newcastle, stopped insisting on the need for notes, and high proportions of the patients were 'casual' or 'emergency'. After treatment ended some dispensaries asked patients to give the subscriber a thank-you note.

Croxson, who studied the late-eighteenth century London dispensaries, concluded that benefactors who supported dispensaries were motivated by social status, fashion, as well as a desire for direct contact with subordinate recipients of charity. The elite figureheads associated with a particular dispensary also contributed to its image, not least because their political affiliation could be used to attract like-minded benefactors. Unlike the publicly acknowledged objectives, these private and political ends provide a clear explanation for the support forthcoming for dispensaries that does not rely on benefactors having an altruistic concern for the needs of the poor.

Fundraising activities of dispensaries included annual charity sermons, preached by prominent clergymen, and usually followed by an anniversary feast. The sermons 'articulated the hopes and motives of the audiences'.[214] Both hospital and dispensary annual reports argued that supporting these institutions benefactors could meet two objectives: those relating directly to curing the sick and those that were purely selfish, such as pleasure or salvation. The dispensaries emphasised that they were less likely than hospitals to engender harmful dependency in recipients and that under some circumstances the type of care offered by a dispensary was more likely to lead to successful treatment.

There were explicit references to three additional sources of personal benefit for dispensary benefactors:

1. Curing the sick poor would prevent the recipients from sinking into pauperism and thereby preventing an increase in the poor rates;
2. Some of the literature maintained that the charity could be a 'passport to heaven';
3. Benefactors were reminded that they might personally benefit from the results of medical research carried out in dispensaries.

The public objectives included

1. the desire to cure – saving lives;
2. a desire to preserve the population for the sake of national wealth and national welfare – a mercantilist-type desire;
3. a type of 'mutual obligation' existing between rich and poor – with the artisan always depending upon the affluent for employment, and the success of the artisan being always necessary to the ease and convenience of the affluent;
4. the requirement that patients abide by the rules was common to all dispensaries – regulations designed to promote social control.

The benefactors faced a choice between supporting hospitals and dispensaries. Publicly, dispensaries maintained that some patients were more likely to be restored to health under their care than that offered by hospitals and some argued that impure air and concomitant danger of infection had a detrimental effect on the health of inpatients. There was also the effect that dispensaries had in reducing the numbers of patients needing to admitted to hospitals. Dispensary literature also mentioned the dangers of 'incarceration' per se, and the detrimental effect of splitting up families.

Some criticised dispensaries as giving too little support and resulted in many supplying patients with food as well as medicine and advice. This, of course, resulted in dispensaries being much less expensive to run than hospitals.

The Private Face of Dispensary Charity

The whole process of recommendations gave benefactors direct contact with the recipients of charity and placed them and the recipients in well-defined roles, as sponsors and suppliants respectively. According to Marland, letters of recommendation acted as a 'conspicuous symbol of the charitable impulses of the rich, and a spur to the gratitude and submission of the poor'.[215]

Benefactions to dispensaries conferred not only the right to recommend patients but also the right to vote for the election of officers.

The aristocratic patrons who served as figureheads also contributed much to the image projected by dispensaries and were consciously sought after. The presence of aristocratic benefactors is consistent with arguments put forward by historians that members of the middle classes advanced their own status by using opportunities offered by voluntary societies to associate with the elite. These opportunities occurred at the general meetings. dispensaries also held annual 'feasts' or festivals.

Volunteers still play an important part in health care in the United Kingdom,[216] especially in hospices, but the role of volunteers in the established health services is diminishing, primarily as a result of the increasing bureaucracy that affects the NHS.

2. An Inexpensive Health Care System

The dispensaries developed because they were economical compared to the cost of running voluntary hospitals and they provided care for those patients too sick to travel to hospitals Loudon[217] suggests that had the voluntary hospitals of the eighteenth and early nineteenth centuries expanded, particularly in the outpatient departments, the dispensaries might never have been founded.

Over the last two centuries various other inexpensive facilities have been created to care for the sick where large hospitals have not provided the care that was needed. Cottage hospitals, homoeopathic hospitals, nursing homes, and hospices have met needs of patients that large hospitals have not been able to meet, and the dispensaries fell into this category. Although most of the dispensaries did not contain beds, they did provide a doctor who would manage patients with illnesses when they couldn't afford traditional medical care.

3. The Dispensaries Managed Many Illnesses Not Admitted to Hospitals

The dispensary doctors looked after many illnesses that would not have been treated in the hospitals.. Infectious diseases were feared by the voluntary hospitals, so if the patient was feverish or had a rash or looked as if he or she might have diarrhoea and/or was vomiting, the patient was viewed with great suspicion and almost certainly not admitted. The last thing the hospital authorities wanted was an outbreak of an infectious disease in the confined situation of a hospital.

Many hospitals stated that young children should not be admitted at all.

4. A Home Visiting Service for Ill People

If a poor person was too weak to leave his or her home, the dispensary doctors would visit to diagnose and treat the problem, provided the patient lived within a carefully circumscribed area around the dispensary and was able to procure a note from a subscriber. If these conditions were not met, the patient had no alternative but to seek help from the Poor Law provision, which after 1834 usually meant receiving admission to a workhouse.

The NHS is often criticised for the reduction in home visiting, but with increasing traffic congestion and difficulty in finding parking places, this is not surprising. Patients nowadays usually have access to their own transport and the wastefulness of doctors sitting in traffic jams means that home visiting is never going to return to levels seen in previous centuries. Nonetheless, there are many calls for patients to receive care at home, particularly during terminal care.

5. A Good Teaching and Research Facility

Many dispensaries became used for teaching purposes, and as we have seen, this occurred mostly in Scotland and the United States of America, where the dispensaries provided medical students with valuable opportunities to learn professional skills. However, following the passing of the Apothecaries Act in 1815, the Society of Apothecaries was able to prescribe a curriculum and insist that those wishing to sit their examination should have attended either a hospital, Infirmary, or dispensary for a period of at least six months.[218] The Society of Apothecaries increased their control on the dispensaries' teaching function over the next few decades by insisting that students should first attend a course of lectures on the principles and practice of medicine, and then that the time spent in the institution should be increased to nine months and that all the physicians attending the dispensary should sign the students' testimony. In 1830 they insisted that attendance at the dispensaries should last for at least fifteen months and that the dispensary should be connected with a medical school that 'was recognised by the court'. This resulted in the creation of fourteen provincial medical schools by 1834.

Cope[219] was able to discover how much teaching resulted from these regulations. During the three years from 1831 to 1833, there were 1,336 candidates for the licentiate examination, of whom 1,171 passed. Of this number there were 222 candidates who had gained their clinical experience in London or at provincial dispensaries, and 193 passed the examination. Fifteen London dispensaries – Islington, Aldersgate Street, The Surrey, St George's and St James. The Western, The South London, The Central, Tower Hamlets, Finsbury, The City, Middlesex, Farringdon, Westminster General, Carey Street, and Bloomsbury – gave instruction.

The provincial dispensaries were York, Wakefield, Salford and Pendleton, Ardwick and Ancoats, Kidderminster, Chorlton, Wigan,

Liverpool North, Leeds, Exeter, Birmingham, Falmouth, Bristol, and Clifton. After 1858 the dispensaries lost their educational function in England and Wales.

The dispensaries made money from teaching, and the fees charged at the St George's and St James's Dispensary, King Street, London, were as follows:

Attendance on the medical establishment for 15 months	6 guineas
Perpetual	8 guineas
Surgical practice 1 year	2 guineas
Perpetual	5 guineas

The Warrington Dispensary library was an unusual development within the dispensaries and was associated with teaching within the dispensary.

Since the 1970s teaching has returned to the community, and departments of general practice are now a key part of the teaching of all medical students in the United Kingdom.[220]

There is little evidence of research being done in dispensaries although William Kay in the Clifton Dispensary used the good record keeping of that dispensary to produce his report on the health of Clifton, an early example of epidemiological research. Robert Willan at the Carey Street Dispensary in London produced much useful early research on skin disease. In 1824 John Forbes described his research using the newly developed stethoscope at the Chichester Dispensary.[221] His cases studies and observations are beautifully described. Before he moved to Chichester in 1822, Forbes was the physician to the Penzance Dispensary, where he had started his research.[222] The earliest research I have found was that of Alexander Gordon's work in Aberdeen on puerperal fever.

6. The Provident Dispensaries

The provident dispensaries appealed to those who believed that the poor value medical services that they have contributed to, and that medical services that are provided at no cost will be abused. Although provident dispensaries increased in numbers at the end of the nineteenth century, they never replaced the voluntary dispensaries totally. Indeed, in Bristol, the provident dispensaries remained small and never appeared to be able to rival the two established voluntary dispensaries. Internationally, there are many examples of 'insurance-based' health systems, such as in the United States and The Netherlands, and many still believe that this provides a more appropriate way of funding health care.

7. Medical Collaboration within Dispensaries

Physicians, surgeons, and apothecaries were all involved with providing medical care within dispensaries. Usually they collaborated well, but there were considerable differences in their responsibilities from one dispensary to another. Physicians such as Dr Lettsom in London, Doctors Ludlow and Chisholm in Bristol, and Dr Dixon in Whitehaven were all the prime instigators in getting dispensaries created in their towns as was the surgeon, Dr Hey in Leeds. The resident medical officers almost always appeared to work well with the physicians and surgeons. There is no doubt that the honorary physicians and surgeons had a much more dominant and frequent presence in some dispensaries such as in Clifton, Exeter, and Greenwich but were less prominent in others, such as Bristol, Liverpool, and Newcastle, where the resident and paid staff did most of the work. It is difficult, though, to know how much work was done by individual doctors as few registers exist.

Much of this collaboration might have been due to the subordinate role that doctors took in the organisation and management of the dispensaries with the subscribers as Governors taking prominent positions on the various dispensary committees. Another reason would be that most doctors in the nineteenth and early twentieth centuries considered themselves generalists rather than specialists and were prepared to deal with all problems presented to them.

8. Charitable Work by Doctors

The vast amount of charitable work done by the nineteenth- and twentieth-century doctors in supporting the dispensaries was remarkable. Even though this free work contributed to the prestige of the doctors and may have increased their income from private patients, few doctors nowadays would consider spending a day working in a clinic for no remuneration, particularly if it involved visiting patients in their homes. This work by doctors was, of course, also supported by much voluntary work by laypeople on the committees of the dispensaries.

Why Did the Dispensaries Fail?

The critical date in the history of the dispensaries in England and Wales was the publication of the Report of the Poor Law Commission in 1907. The majority report of this commission described the free dispensaries in the following way[223]:

> One striking feature brought out as the result of our enquiries into the methods of providing poor persons with medical assistance is the existence in certain large urban centres of extensive free dispensaries, while in another centre, with not dissimilar industrial conditions, such dispensaries are practically, if not entirely, absent. Thus, on the one hand, we have in towns as Birmingham, Leeds, and Newcastle flourishing free dispensaries. The Newcastle Dispensary, we are informed, does the greater part of the outdoor medical work for the poor of the city. It has seven whole-time doctors; it treats about twelve thousand patients per annum; and, as compared with the Poor Law, it does ten or twenty times as much work among the poor. On the other hand, Sheffield has no free dispensary, and Leicester is mainly served by

215

provident dispensaries. There are, it may be observed, a number of free dispensaries in London.

The quality of the treatment at the dispensaries is said to be of a high order, and this, together with the fact that it is free, attracts large numbers of persons to apply. In some dispensaries treatment is mainly confined to persons who produce a subscriber's ticket, but in others no tickets are necessary.

Our evidence clearly shows that the benefits of free dispensaries are abused by many who could well afford to pay ordinary fees to a doctor. Witnesses have told us that the free dispensaries are powerful and successful competitors of the Provincial dispensaries and the medical clubs and operate with hardship on the medical profession.

The majority report recommended[224]:

That a general system of provident dispensaries should be established of which existing voluntary outdoor medical organisations be invited to form an integral part, and that every inducement should be offered to the working classes below a certain wage limit to become, or to continue to be, members of a provident dispensary. To this end, the subscription to the provident dispensary should cover the following advantages to its members:

1. power to choose their own doctor from the doctors upon the list of the dispensary;

2. the provision of adequate medical assistance at a rate or fee within the reach of those subscribing to the provident dispensary;

3. institutional treatment upon a recommendation from the dispensary doctor

The Views of the Minority Report

The minority report, written largely by Sidney and Beatrice Webb, saw the dispensaries in a very different light[225]:

> It has been represented to us that the whole provision for the sick now made by the Destitution Authority, alike in its domiciliary treatment and in its 'hospital branch', is but the fringe of a more general provision for the sick made by other agencies; that these other agencies impinge upon the medical work of the Poor Law and are themselves impeded by it; and that if the Poor Law medical work were brought to an end or seriously restricted, they might with advantage undertake the whole service. These voluntary agencies in some cases provide their services gratuitously; others claim to be self-supporting; whilst others again exact a partial contribution for their benefits. Across this classification runs the cleavage between those voluntary agencies maintaining residential institutions and those supplying only domiciliary treatment.
>
> To begin with the domiciliary treatment of the sick poor, we find the overlapping work of the district medical officer,

1. the Free Dispensary or 'medical mission';

2. the outpatient department of the voluntary hospital;

3. the doctor's medical club or the Friendly Society or other 'contract practice';

4. the medical provident association started by a combination of local doctors or the provident dispensary managed by a philanthropic committee.

These four classes of agencies for domiciliary treatment of the sick poor differ widely from one another in their geographical extension, the doctor's medical club or contract practice being, for instance, widespread over town and country alike, and the outpatients' department being confined to the metropolis and a few large towns. They differ also in the degree to which, in one place or another, they impinge upon or overlap the Poor Law.

The Free Dispensaries and 'medical missions', on the one hand, and the outpatients' departments of the voluntary hospitals on the other, have in common the attribute of offering medical attendance and medicine gratuitously to those who come for it at prescribed times and places – sometimes without the slightest fee or formality, sometimes on presentation of a subscriber's letter, and sometimes on payment of a few pence for the medicine supplied. Started originally on a small scale ... these centres of gratuitous doctoring now minister ... to literally hundreds of thousands of cases annually. The vast outpatient departments of the voluntary hospitals, with their ever open doors, offering gratuitous treatment to all comers, are a standing obstacle to any efficient reform of the home treatment of the sick poor. What is more serious is the assertion that the treatment afforded to the bulk of patients is, from the standpoint of preventive or really curative treatment, wholly unsatisfactory.

We need not describe the Free Dispensaries and 'medical missions' which abound in the slum districts of a few large towns. All the arguments about the gratuitous, indiscriminate, and unconditional medical attendance by the outpatients' departments of the hospitals appear to us to apply, in even greater strength, to the Free Dispensaries and medical missions'; with the added drawbacks, they are not, as a rule, under responsible and specialised medical supervision, and that they are not able to offer immediate institutional treatment to those that require it.

In a contemporary publication,[226] the Webbs' report the comment of 'an experienced physician' about dispensary doctors:

[T]hey give people a bottle of medicine, but they do not do much else. They take no supervision of their home surroundings, and no supervision of the general hygiene, and they never provide anything in the way of food and nourishment. It is very often much more food that is wanted, for instance, with the children.

They added that 'the medical practitioner who is chary with drugs, but prodigal and plainspoken in his advice about giving up bad habits and drinking, is seldom popular among the poor'.

Not surprisingly, the authors of the minority report had very different conclusions and recommendations[227]:

After careful consideration of the working and results of medical insurance [club practices and Friendly

Societies], our conclusion is that we should hesitate before recommending these. All provident clubs and dispensary practice fail in that they give people a bottle of medicine, but they do not do much else. They take no supervision of their home surroundings and no supervision of the general hygiene, and they never provide anything in the way of food and nourishment. We believe it is quite impossible to employ any system of medical insurance as a substitute for the Poor Law Medical Service.

It has been suggested that the Provident Medical Associations be fortified by a compulsory enactment, requiring every adult to become a member for himself and his dependants. The short answer to this suggestion is that in this country, under present conditions, it is totally impracticable. To bring the government to collect weekly contributions from hundreds of thousands of unskilled and casually employed labourers would be an impossible task. Such collections would be in the nature of a poll tax and England has not had a poll tax since 1381. The government would also have to guarantee the management – a task of gigantic dimensions.

The most serious objection is that, in the treatment of poor persons, the problem is complicated by the frequent necessity for supplementing the medical attendance by 'medical extras' – that is to say nourishing food and stimulants of one sort or another. Doctors would be under pressure to provide such 'extras', and this would interfere with their medical treatments.

The authors of the minority report disagreed with the recommendations in the majority report[228]:

With regard to the suggestion that the medical treatment of the sick poor should be left either to provident medical insurance or to voluntary charity, it has been demonstrated to us that these offer no possible alternative to the provision for the sick made by the public authority. We disagree with the suggestion that the poor should choose their own doctor – this would ensure that there would be extravagant expenditure on popular remedies and 'medical extras'. The need is for a unified medical service in which the medical services of the Poor Law and the Public Health Authorities would be merged. A public health service would change the approach of medicine from a curative service to a preventive one.

As Cope[229] has written, if ever the dispensary system had become the basis of a national health service as was quite a possibility following the majority report of the Poor Law commission, then the number of dispensaries would have had to be substantially increased, the whole population would have had to be compelled to join one or other type of dispensary and with large state subsidies added to the weekly contribution of each member (or poll tax, as the minority report called it), there would have been ample funds available to pay all the doctors who wanted to join the scheme. As it was, the views of the members of the minority report prevailed and the development and expansion of the dispensaries ceased.

Sidney and Beatrice Webb believed that the provision of a free medical service by compulsory health insurance would ultimately 'demoralize' both the medical profession and the public; doctors would try every means to lure patients into their surgeries at the state's expense. And the gullible working class would take to medicine as it had already taken to drink. What was needed was a neat, efficient system of environmental services.[230]

Some Conclusions

Medicine has changed in many ways since the dispensaries started appearing. Over the last two hundred years there have been remarkable developments:

- In Britain it is now normal for people to live to 100 years;
- The commonest causes of death are now those associated with blood vessel diseases and cancers rather than infections.
- Surgeons commonly replace worn-out joints and worn-out organs such as kidneys, livers, and even hearts and lungs.
- There is much emphasis on prevention of disease: immunisations against most of the infectious diseases, advice, and medicines reduce the risk of blood vessel disease.
- Most elderly people take regular medication in order to keep in good health.
- It is rare for children to die in infancy, and many premature babies grow normally.
- A high proportion of the population live with allergies to popular foodstuffs.
- Everybody is registered with a primary-care doctor who retains a computerised medical record of all their health problems.
- Most doctors working outside hospitals now work in groups of more than three with many supporting staff and in purpose built premises, and in the United Kingdom these doctors are responsible for the medical care of all their registered patients.
- Doctors have to carry medical indemnity insurance as any mistake is likely to result in a lawsuit with significant financial penalties.
- Evidence-based medicine and guidelines for management of conditions have been developed and instituted as key parts of the health service.

Since the government started running the NHS, doctors and other health service staff have found themselves increasingly controlled in attempts to improve quality, reduce costs and respond to political initiatives. Every new administration believes they know how to improve the NHS and often institute change with little experimental evidence to back their views. Successive governments believe that doctors must be accountable for the work they do and have introduced extensive and threatening bodies like the Care Quality Commission to achieve this. The contrast with the largely 'hands-off' management of dispensaries is obvious.

I don't believe the dispensaries provided an excellent system of health care – the care the doctors in dispensaries provided certainly fell far short of what the National Health Service provides now, but dispensary care does point to many ways in which the health service could be improved. It also provides us with many opportunities to rethink the way we run our NHS.

How about these challenges?

- Why do we retain the right of everybody to access acute health care without cost, when almost everybody is prepared to spend several hundreds of pounds on a television set, a holiday, and alcohol? Many pay similar amounts on season tickets for football matches. I can understand the need to provide free health care for expensive essential operations, investigations and cancer treatment, but a consultation with a doctor is not, nowadays, very expensive. Patients who are receiving state benefits or who have chronic diseases that require regular monitoring should be excused from paying for consultations – but surely not the rest. Providing a financial barrier to that initial consultation is also likely to help reduce the frequency of consultations for minor respiratory infections and the consequent reduction in the request for antibiotics.
- Why do we continue to freely provide preventive medicine, such as blood pressure-reducing tablets, cholesterol-lowering

medication, and such to people over the age of say, 80, when their quality of life is poor?

- Why doesn't the NHS fund hospices? After all, they provide terminal care with great skill and are considered an essential part of health care. Currently, their main source of funds is from charitable giving.

- Why don't we have regionally appointed lay-groups with medical support to make decisions about health care for people with rare conditions and to decide on priorities in health care provision? Using volunteers in this way is likely to bring back the best of the dispensary management system. The old community health councils provided a necessary check on the health services.

There will be many other ideas that the dispensary story will stimulate – after all, people involved in the dispensaries gained much satisfaction from their jobs and were able to achieve much. Many patients received excellent care and were grateful for it.

Rudolf Klein[231] has emphasised the enormous social, environmental, and political changes that have taken place since the NHS came into being. He considers that the authors of the NHS saw it as paternalistic, meeting needs and requiring planning. It would answer most needs, even though it would require the creation of priorities, and above all, would expect trust in and from its staff. He claims that the NHS has now evolved to become like a garage, where the demands of consumerism and responsiveness are centred on contracts; professional providers can no longer be trusted to be selfless altruists; patients must have choice, but they must also take on responsibility for ensuring their bodies remain healthy. As Klein has stated: 'The vocabulary of the market – choice and competition – has become the language of policy debate. Deference to medical authority is no longer automatic as the patient, reborn as a consumer, shops on the web'.

James McCormick, in his book *The Doctor, Father Figure, or Plumber*,[232] quotes Sir George Pickering as saying that medicine is at a crossroads, having chosen the downhill road where a learned profession will ultimately be reduced to a technological trade union. McCormick, however, suggests that medicine can combine technical competence with knowledge of its limitations; it is possible to recognise human needs and to allow to Everyman his autonomy and his right to human dignity. This demands more than knowledge of disease; it demands concern and awareness of people as individual, unique, human beings.

Dr Howard Stoate wrote in 2015,[233]

> I have been a GP for nearly thirty-five years and am heading towards retirement. I have just stepped down from chairing a clinical commissioning group after a five-year term. A GP friend who has taken early retirement, simply due to pressure of work, asked me the other day: 'Who will be my GP when I am old and frail?' It is a good question. Being a GP is a wonderful and privileged career, and by any standards it is well paid. So why does no one want to do it anymore? Even 'good' practices cannot recruit, and many are reaching crisis point, with the real threat of closures.
>
> General practice is facing a perfect storm. The proportion of NHS spending allocated to primary care has fallen steadily. It is now around 7 per cent, and with this we deal with 90 per cent of patient contacts. Our population is ageing. Older people have more health problems, and need more time. We are constantly under pressure to reduce the number of referrals, hospital admissions, A&E attendances, and prescribing levels. Patients are becoming better informed and quite rightly expect more from their NHS. Everyone needs a bigger slice of a cake which, at best, is the same size as it was five years ago. General practitioners take the brunt of this pressure;

young doctors coming out of medical school look on with dismay and are simply not prepared to take it on.

The government cannot be unaware of this situation, but its response is to promise five thousand 'new' GPs by 2020 (where from?), in return for routine GP appointments available twelve hours a day, seven days a week. Is it cock-up, or something more sinister? It all reminds me of the story of the farmer who, faced with financial problems, came up with a cunning plan. Over many months, he painstakingly trained his donkey to eat less and less food. Just as it was getting used to eating nothing at all, it died.

Sidney and Beatrice Webb, in the preface of their book *The State and the Doctor*,[234] written at the beginning of the twentieth century, wrote, 'We owe it to the doctors not to hamper their beneficent work by clumsy administrative organisation. We can, at any rate, stand out of their way; and this, at present, we are not doing'.

For most people illness is episodic, requiring, after self-care and discussion with others, the help of a health professional who is easily available. This doctor or nurse must have a broad training and have good communication skills and the knowledge to refer to an appropriate specialist if necessary – not much different from the dispensary system, except that we now have much easier access to care, incredibly clever treatments and the ability to improve much chronic ill-health.

APPENDIX

THE DEVELOPMENT OF THE MEDICAL PROFESSION IN THE UNITED KINGDOM

Throughout this book the word 'doctor' has included the professional term of physician, surgeon, apothecary, general practitioner, and medical officer. During the last three centuries these types of doctor have worked in dispensaries, and in order to understand the relationship between the medical profession and the dispensary, it is necessary to understand the significance of these words.

The Physician

In the mid-eighteenth century physicians were regarded, and certainly thought of themselves, as the most learned and socially superior class of practitioner. They usually entered the profession through an apprenticeship and then studied and took their doctorate of medicine at a university. In England, Oxford and Cambridge were the only two universities, and most aspirants for the degree studied in Scotland, principally in Edinburgh or Glasgow, or went to Europe, for example to the universities of Paris, Leyden, and Pisa. They practised internal medicine and in effect treated their patients by giving advice and prescribing medicines which were then made up by apothecaries who charged for their dispensing services and drugs but were not legally allowed to give advice to patients or themselves to prescribe. The College of Physicians was founded in 1518 in London and the Edinburgh College of Physicians in 1681.

Apothecaries

Apothecaries were trained by apprenticeship, sometimes in a Society of Apothecaries, as in London, but in others in a Grocers or Spicers Company.

The Surgeon

Few surgeons took a degree of doctor of medicine. The great majority were members of surgeons or barber-surgeons guilds and were admitted after five years' apprenticeship with a practising surgeon. By 1750 surgeons were practically separate from those of barbers. Surgeons, in effect, looked after the outside of the body treating injuries, dislocations, and fractures and performing amputations. They also operated on superficial tumours, opened abscesses, and treated ulcers and other skin conditions. Some specialised in removing bladder stones. Surgeons were not legally permitted to prescribe internal medicines for their patients. But these rules, like those relating to apothecaries, were commonly ignored, and surgeons did general practice as did apothecaries for the great mass of people.

During the nineteenth century the position changed completely. The College of Surgeons in London, founded in 1800, received the Royal Charter in 1824 and began to hold examinations for membership. Nine years earlier, the Apothecaries Act made the Licence of the London Society of Apothecaries a requirement for practice in England. The examinations of both institutions were held in London, and candidates had to submit certificates showing that they had attended approved lecture courses. Both institutions recognised the provincial medical schools that were created in the early part of the century, as appropriate places to receive such training. The Certificate of the Membership of the College of Surgeons (MRCS) and the License of the Society of Apothecaries (LSA) became the recognised qualifications for general practice and remained so until the universities initiated their own medical degrees in the second half of the century.

In 1858 the Medical Act was passed. This established the medical register and identified the bodies whose teaching or examinations would be recognised for the purpose of enrolment in the medical register, without which it was not legal to practise medicine. During the same period the Royal Colleges of Surgeons and Physicians in London instituted examinations for those who wished to be recognised as surgeons or physicians whether or not they were in general practice.

The twentieth century has seen the development of the medical specialities where physicians and surgeons have restricted their work and expertise to limited areas of the body or type of practice. So we now have paediatricians, obstetricians, gynaecologists, pathologists, radiologists, and so on, and each of these specialities has developed their own college, training requirements, and examinations. These clinical specialists now restrict their work mostly to within major hospitals although other specialists such as occupational health specialists, public health specialists and some psychiatrists work outside these institutions.

ABOUT THE AUTHOR

Dr Whitfield is a retired Bristol general practitioner who was a senior lecturer in general practice in the University of Bristol. He has been writing about the history of medicine over the last ten years. His recent publications have included *The Victorian Doctors of Victoria Square* (2011) and *A Short History of Academic General Practice in the UK Medical Schools 1948–2000* (with John Howie, 2011).

ABOUT THE BOOK

Dispensaries were created in cities to look after poor, sick people from about 1770 until the beginning of the NHS in 1948. They were created by relatively wealthy citizens who became subscribers to these institutions. They saw this as an act of philanthropy, and each subscriber was given a book of tickets that could be given to sick people to enable them to access the dispensary. Many doctors gave their services to the dispensaries freely, but an apothecary or later on a medical officer was employed to run the dispensary and to visit the sick in their homes if necessary.

This is the first book to give an overview of the creation of dispensaries and the reason they disappeared by 1948. The dispensary system was supported by the majority report of the Royal Commission on the Poor Law in 1909 but rejected on questionable grounds by the minority report, upon which our welfare state has been based.

Currently, the NHS is in crisis, and this book about a former health care system suggests ways in which our health service could be remodelled for the better.

REFERENCES

BMJ is British Medical Journal
BRO is Bristol Record Office

1   Z Cope, *A Forgotten Health Service, Being the Story of the General Medical Dispensaries in Britain*. Unpublished book, London: Wellcome Library, 1966.

2   I Loudon, 'The Origins and Growth of the Dispensary Movement in England', *Bulletin of the History of Medicine*, 55 (1981) 322–42.

3   RG Hodgkinson, *The Origins of the National Health Service*, London: The Wellcome Historical Medical Library, 1967, 303.

4   M Fissell, 'Patients, Power, and the Poor in Eighteenth-Century Bristol', *Cambridge History of Medicine* (1991).

5   AW Hill, *John Wesley among the Physicians*, London: The Epworth Press, 1958, 47.

6   Loudon, 322–42.

7   T Beddoes, 'Considerations on Infirmaries, 1791' in *Memoirs of the Life of Thomas Beddoes John Edmunds Stock 1811*, London: John Murrary.

8   D Stansfield, *Thomas Beddoes MD 1760–1808*. D Reidel Publishing Company, 1914, 184.

9   *An account of the Bristol Dispensary*, 1776, BRO 40442/72.

10   Biographical Memoirs, 11, 566, BRO 35893/36/n.

11   Ibid.

12   JO Symes, *A Short History of Bristol General Hospital*, Bristol: John Wright and Sons Ltd, 1932, 8.

13   RG Hodgkinson, 191.

14   Ibid., 270.

15   G Wallis, Free Medical Aid to the Poor without Pauperism in Lieu of the Present Method of Poor Law Medical Relief http://www.jstor.org/stable/60249868. Accessed 14.11.15.

16   M Whitfield, *The Bristol Microscopists and the Cholera Epidemic of 1849,* ALHA book, No 9, 2011.

17   *British Medical Journal,* 19 Jan 1855, 65.

18   www.workhouses.org.uk/ireland/; accessed 20.12.2014.

19   RG Hodgkinson, 694.

20   FJ Fry, 'On the Opening of the New Dispensary', *Bristol Mercury and Daily Post,* 11 July 1888.

21   'Lest You Forget No 50 Anon', *Western Daily Press* and *Bristol Mirror,* 30 September 1942.

22   Loudon, 322–42.

23   Dresser M., ed. *The Diary of Sarah Fox* 2003, Bristol Record Office, 43.

24   Ibid.

25   JP Bush, 'Early History of the Bristol Royal Infirmary', *Bristol Med Chi J* (Sept 1908), 205.

26   G Munro Smith, *History of the Bristol Royal Infirmary,* Bristol: Arrowsmith, 1917, 118.

27   M Dresser, 25.

28   Bristol Record Office, Biographical Memoirs No 14, 35893/36/n., 227.

29   Loudon, 322–42.

30   JC Prichard, *A History of the Epidemic Fever, Which Prevailed in Bristol during ... 1817, 1818, and 1819,* Nabu Press, 2011.

31   Bristol Record Office, 19244/7.

32   Letter to *The Lancet.* 1 (1845), 218.

33   *The Bristol Mercury,* May 5, 1849.

34   *The Bristol Mercury,* 19 October 1861.

35   *The Bristol Mercury,* 14 January 1886.

36   *The Bristol Mercury,* 25 November 1876.

37   *Bristol Mercury* and *Daily Post,* 3 January 1879.

38   *Bristol Mercury* and *Daily Post,* 8 January 1880.

39   FJ Fry, 'On the Opening of the New Dispensary', *Bristol Mercury and Daily Post,* 11 July 1888.

40   Plans of Castle Green Dispensary, BRO.plan/vol22/2a

41   Bristol Dispensary Annual Report, 1854, Bristol Reference Library.

42   Bristol Record Office 33041 BMC/13/1-4.

43   CEK Herepath, 'Auricular Fibrillation', *Bristol Med-Chi J,* 29 (1911), 148–50.

44   Bristol Dispensary Minutes, Bristol Record Office 33041 BMC/13/1–4, 21 September 1906.

45   Bristol Record Office 33041 BMC/13/1–4, 11 January 1907.

46   Bristol Record Office 33041 BMC/13/1-4.

47   CB Perry, *The Voluntary Medical Institutions of Bristol,* No 56 Bristol Branch of the Historical Association, The University, 1984.

48   Bristol Record Office 33041, 639.

49   CB Perry, 8.

50   C Chisholm, 'On the Statistical Pathology of Bristol and of Clifton, Gloucestershire', *The Edinburgh Medical and Surgical Journal* (1 July 1817), 266.

51   MR Neve, *Natural Philosophy, Medical, and Other Cultural Sciences in Provincial England,* PhD thesis, London: University College, 1984.

52   Biographical Memoirs, 11, 566, BRO 35893/36/k

53   Report of the General Meeting of the Subscribers of the Clifton Dispensary December 1 1812, Bristol Reference Library

54   MI Lattimore *Journal of the Royal Naval Medical Service,* 67 (summer 1981), 92.

55   *Medico-Chirurgical Journal,* 2 (1819–20), 104.

56   Lavars BRO 40556.

57   Plarr's Lives of the Fellows Online Royal College Surgeons, accessed 2014.

58   M Whitfield, *Dr Goodeve and Cook's Folly.* ALHA books, No 4, 2010.

59   *The London Gazette,* 23 September 1845, 2918.

60   G Munro Smith, *A History of the Bristol Royal Infirmary.* Bristol: Arrowsmith, 1917, 304.

61   *The London Gazette,* 8 February 1828, 281.

62   W Kay, *The Sanitary Condition of Bristol and Clifton* (Bristol 1844).

63   *Bristol Mercury* and *Daily Post* March 10 1855.

64   *Bristol Mercury* and *Daily Post* Sept 12 1857.

65   BRO 39801/F/20.

66   G Munro Smith, 450.

67   *Bristol Mercury* and *Daily Post* Feb 6 1878.

68   *Bristol Mercury* and *Daily Post* Feb 5 1879.

69   *Bristol Mercury* and *Daily Post* Feb 7 1894.

70   Clifton Dispensary Minute Book BRO 33041/bmc/13/5.

71   Obituary, *Bristol Med-Chi J,* 53 (1935), 85.

72   Biographical Memoirs, 7 BRO, 35893/36/g.

73   Marmion V *The Bristol Eye Hospital Bristol* Medico-Historical Society 2010, 24.

74   G Munro Smith A *History of the Bristol Royal Infirmary,* Arrowsmith Bristol 1917.

75   Matthews Bristol Directory 1860. published by Matthew Matthews London 362

76   *Bristol Mercury* and *Daily Post*, 29 April 1896.

77   Matthews Directory 1890.

78   *Bristol Mercury*, 22 October 1838.

79   Matthews Directory 1840.

80   *London Medical Gazette*, 27 (1840), 223.

81   Biographical Memoirs 7 BRO 35893/36/g.

82   G Munro Smith *A History of the Bristol Royal Infirmary,* Bristol: Arrowsmith, 1917, 192.

83   Biographical Memoirs 12 BRO 35893/36/l.

84   *Daily Post*, 10 April 1867.

85   Plarr's Lives of the Surgeons online at www.rcseng.ac.uk, accessed 2015.

86   Matthews Directory 1870.

87   Biographical Memoirs 14 BRO 35893/36/n.

88   Biographical Memoirs 14 BRO 35893/36/n.

89   Matthew's Directory 1853.

90   Bartley RTF *The Lancet*, 48 (1846), 32, 172, and 237.

91   CD Evans, 'A History of Dermatology in Bristol and the West of England', *Br J Derm*, 86 (1972), 180.

92   BRI Faculty: Minutes, Bristol Record Office 1876.

93   O Wunderlich, 'The Work of the Metropolitan Provident Medical Association', *BMJ,* (6 March 1897), 603.

94   G Munro Smith, 400.

95   S Cordery, *British Friendly Societies 1750–1914,* Palgrave Macmillan, 2003, 105.

96   *Bristol Mercury* and *Daily Post*, 9 June 1888.

97   P Gosden, The Friendly Societies in England 1815–1875.

98   S Cordery, 142.

99   *Bristol Mercury*, 27 June 1874.

100   *Bristol Mercury* and *Daily Post*, 22 October 1883.

101   *British Medical Journal*, 6 January 1917, 35.

102   Wright's Directory, Bristol 1910.

103   Bristol Medical Missionary Society 25th Anniversary Annual Report 1897, Bristol Reference Library B35132.

104   WF Mack, 'Occasional Paper of the Bristol Medical Mission Bristol 1897', Bristol Reference Library B35132.

105   M Whitfield, *Homoeopathy in Bristol 1840–1925*, ALHA Books No 15.

106   M Gorsky, *Patterns of Philanthropy*, Royal Historical Press, 1999, 157.

107   *Bristol Mercury* and *Daily Post*, 14 March 1868.

108   Matthews Directory, 1900, 739.

109   *Bristol Mercury*, February 1862.

110   *The Times*, 11 May 1878.

111   Matthews Directory 1900.

112   *Bristol Mercury*, 1896.

113   W Hartston, 'Medical Dispensaries in Eighteenth-Century London', Proceedings of the Royal College of Medicine, 56 (1963), 753–8.

114   JC Lettsom, Medical Memoires of the General Dispensary in London. Edward and Charles Dilley 1774

115   RG Hodgkinson, *The origins of the National Health Service,* The Wellcome Historical Medical Library, 1967, 206.

116   R Richardson, Lettsom's morning walk *The Lancet*, 359 (27 April 2002), 1530.

117   Hartston, 757.

118   Ibid., 757.

119   J Millar *Observations on the Practice in the Medical Department of the Westminster General Dispensary* London 1777.

120   *The Chemist and Druggist*, 29 June 1957.

121   *Rules, Orders, and Regulations of the Surrey Dispensary* J Robins and Sons, Southwark 1822

122   *The Lancet*, 143 (1894), 1023.

123   Ibid., 1098.

124 Ibid., 1274.

125 J Poland, *Records of the Miller Hospital and Royal Kent Dispensary,* Greenwich: H Richardson, 1893.

126 Poland, 41

127 Loudon, 327.

128 M Sydney, *Bleeding, Blisters, and Opium: Joshua Dixon and the Whtehaven Dispensary.* Workington: Stainburn Publications, 2009.

129 *British Medical Journal,* 14 August, 1897, 411.

130 R Ridley-Smith, *The New Zealand Medical Journal,* 119, no 1233 (2006), 90.

131 H MacCormac, 'At the Public Dispensary with Willan and Bateman'. *The British Journal of Dermatology and Syphilis,* XLV (October 1933), 385–95.

132 *Plan of the Public Dispensary, Carey Street,* e-book, Wellcome Library.

133 A Swank, A Grzybowski, and LC Parish, *Clinics in Dermatology,* 29 (2001), 567–70.

134 R McAuliffe *The Story of the Bloomsbury Dispensary,* The Trustees of the Bloomsbury Dispensary, 1973, 6–7.

135 McAuliffe, 8.

136 NH Schuster, *The Western General Dispensary,* St Marylebone Society Publication No. 5, 1961.

137 Schuster, 8.

138 Schuster, 25.

139 Report of the Royal Commission on the Poor Laws Vol 1. Her Majesty's Stationery Office London, 1909, 321.

140 SC Lawrence, *Charitable Knowledge, Hospital Pupils, and Practitioners in Eighteenth-Century London,* Cambridge History of Medicine, 1996, 41.

141 R Bogle, *From Charity to Providence: Influences on the Organisation of Dispensaries in the Early Nineteenth Century,* 2012 Diploma in the History of Medicine. Society of Apothecaries.

142 Hodgkinson, 212.

143 The Medical Directory 1875 John Churchill and Sons, London

144 Loudon, 323.

145 Stevens Pauline *Stroud Dispensary* http://www.stroudlocalhistorysociety.org.uk/research/Dispensary/, accessed July 2015.

146   R Guest-Gornall, *The Warrington Dispensary Library. Medical History*, 11 (July 1967), 285–96.

147   M Sydney, *Bleeding, Blisters, and Opium: Joshua Dixon and the Whtehaven Dispensary*. Workington: Stainburn Publications, 2009.

148   Loudon, 339.

149   History written by HT, 22 December 1952 from the South Dispensary 1, Upper Parliament Street, Liverpool D627/1 Special Collections; Liverpool University Library.

150   Report of the Committee of the Liverpool Dispensaries 1838 D274 Special Collections; Liverpool University Library.

151   Hodgkinson, 208.

152   Letter from Michael Sheridan FRCS D627/2 Special Collections; Liverpool University Library.

153   EC Bosworth, *Public Health Care in Nottingham 1750 to 1911,* PhD Thesis submitted to University of Nottingham May 1998.

154   J Storer, *Hints on the Constitution of Dispensaries,* London: J Hatchard & Son, 1832, 13–14.

155   www.ancoatsdispensarytrust.co.uk, accessed November 2015.

156   H Marland, 'Lay and Medical Conceptions of Medical Charity during the Nineteenth Century in Medicine and Charity before the Welfare State', Barry J and Jones C Routledge, eds, London and New York, 1991, 150.

157   Marland, 159.

158   J Wilmot, Thesis, Oxford University, 2014.

159   Dorset History Centre NG/CC: P38/1.

160   *The Lancet,* 9 December 1905, 1733.

161   Minute Book of the Dispensary 1905 Devon Heritage Centre G1/F34

162   Temporary Catalogue, compiled by Joyce Percy, York City Archives, 1960s amendments and additions, Katherine Webb, 2013www.york.ac.uk/borthwick.

163   GA Butler, *Disease, Medicine, and the Urban Poor in Newcastle-upon-Tyne, c. 1750–1850.* PhD thesis, Newcastle University, January 2012.

164   Butler, 304.

165   Butler, 2.

166   DM Thomson, 'General Practice and the Edinburgh Medical School', *Journal Royal College of General Practitioners*, 34 (1984), 9–12.

167   DA Sutton, *The Public-Private Interface of Domiciliary Medical Care for the Poor in Scotland c. 1875–1911,* PhD thesis University of Glasgow, November 2009, 164.

168   Sutton, 169.

169   *The Lancet,* 23 August 1898, 418.

170   Z Cope, 'The influence of the Free Dispensaries upon Medical Education', *Medical History*, 13.1 (1969), 36.

171   Sutton, 195.

172   C Cameron, Glasgow Medical Missionary Society Annual Report (1883), 7.

173   Sutton, 182.

174   Bennett PN Alexander Gordon (1752–99) and His Writing: Insights into Medical Thinking in the Late Eighteenth Century', *J R Coll Physicians Edinb,* 42 (2012), 165–71.

175   RD Cassell, *Medical Charities, Medical Politics The Irish Dispensary System and the Poor Law 1836–72,* The Royal Historical Society, Boydell Press, 1997, 8.

176   GM Beale, 'Dispensaries in Counties Armagh and Down in the Pre-Famine Years', *The Ulster Medical Journal*, 66 No 2 (1997), 123–33.

177   Cassell, 92.

178   Beale, 123–33.

179   P Starr, *The Social Transformation of American Medicine,* New York: Basic Books, 1949, 182.

180   CE Rosenburg, 'Social Class and Medical Care in Nineteenth-Century America: the Rise and Fall of the Dispensary', *Journal of the History of Medicine* (January 1974), 32–54.

181   Rosenburg, 34.

182   Ibid. 36.

183   MM Davis and AR Warner, *Dispensaries: Their Management and Development*, New York: The Macmillan Co, 1918, 38.

184   The Rules and By-Laws of the Baltimore General Dispensary 1803 Baltimore.

185   Starr, 183.

186   Rosenburg, 47.

187 'Status and Standards of Dispensary Practice', *California State Journal of Medicine,* XIV, no 12 (1916), 487.

188 Starr, 182.

189 Rosenburg, 53.

190 *Sydney Herald,* 1 May 1840.

191 *Sydney Morning Herald,* 6 February 1850.

192 J Blake, *The Dispensary Movement in Bombay Presidency: Ideology and Practice 1800–75* Master of Philosophy thesis School of Oriental and African Studies 2004.

193 M Harrison, *Public Health in British India: Anglo-Indian Preventive Medicine,* Cambridge University Press, 1994.

194 D.Arnold, *Colonising the body; state medicine and epidemics disease in nineteenth century India.* University of California Press 1999, 273.

195 Projit Bihari Mukharji, 'Structuring Plurality: Locality, Caste, Class, and Ethnicity in Nineteenth-Century Bengali Dispensaries', *Health and History,* 9, no 1 (2007), 80–105.

196 AB Granville, *A Report of the Practice of Midwifery at the Westminster General Dispensary,* London Burgess and Hill, 1818.

197 J Storer. *Hints on the Constitution of Dispensaries,* London: J Hatchard & Son, 1832.

198 AP Stewart, *Sanitary Economics,* 1850.

199 HL Smith, 'Provident Dispensaries: Their Social Importance and Their Advantages to the Medical Profession', *London Journal Medicine,* s2-2 (1850), 368–75.

200 Hodgkinson, 614.

201 G Munro Smith, 315.

202 G Rivett, *The Development of the London Hospital System;* see www.nhshistory.net.

203 Symes, 49.

204 Symes, 49.

205 JF Anderson, 'Provident Dispensaries: Their Object and Practical Working', *BMJ* (21 May 1870), 516.

206 *The Times,* 27 April 1882.

207 O Wunderlich, 'The Work of the Metropolitan Provident Medical Association', *BMJ* (6 March 1897), 603.

208 R Bogle, *From Charity to Providence: Influences on the Organisation of Dispensaries in the Early Nineteenth Century',*

thesis for the diploma in the History of Medicine Society of Apothecaries, 2012.

209   J Wilmot, 'Advice and Medicine for the Working Classes: The Leamington and Warwick Provident Dispensaries 1869–1913', *Warwickshire History*, XV, no 1 (2014), 26–42.

210   J Jones, *Self-Supporting Dispensaries*, London: John Churchill, 1862.

211   *British Medical Association*, 8 June 1895, 1271.

212   S Heydon, *The provision of medical care for the poor in Leicester in the 1830s* Leicester Archaeological and Historical Society, 55 (1979–80), 70.

213   M Prentice, *The Firth Provident Medical Dispensary*. Vale and Downland Museum Trust, 1987.

214   B Croxson, 'The Public and Private Faces of Eighteenth-Century London Dispensary Charity', *Medical History*, 41 (1997), 127–49.

215   H Marland, *Medicine and Society in Wakefield and Huddersfield, 1780–1870*, Cambridge University Press, 1987.

216   C Mundle, C Naylor, and D Buck, *Volunteering in Health and Care in England: A Summary of Key Literature*, King's Fund, July 2012.

217   Loudon, 322–42.

218   Z Cope, "The Influence of the Free Dispensaries upon Medical Education in Britain," *Medical History* 13 (1969) 29–36.

219   Ibid., 33–4.

220   J Howie and M Whitfield, *Academic General Practice in the UK Medical Schools 1948-2000*, Edinburgh University Press, 2011.

221   J Forbes, *Original Cases with Dissections and Observations Illustrating the Stethoscope and Percussion in the Diagnosis of Diseases of the Chest*. London: T. & G. Underwood, 1824.

222   Craig, John. "A General Dispensary Practice 150 Years Ago," *Aberdeen University Review* 44 no. 148 (1972) 358–67.

223   Report of the Royal Commission on the Poor Laws Vol 1. Her Majesty's Stationery Office, London, 1909, 335.

224   Ibid., 264.

225   B Webb and S Webb, eds., *Break-Up of the Poor Law, Being Part One of the Minority Report of the Poor Law Commission*, London: Longmans, Green, and Co. 1909, 249.

226   B Webb and S Webb, *The State and the Doctor*, London: Longmans, Green, and Co. 1910, 144.

227   Minority Report, 258.

228   Ibid., 291.

229   Z Cope, *A Forgotten Health Service, Being the Story of the General Medical Dispensaries in Britain*. Unpublished book, London: Wellcome Library, 1966.

230   S Webb, *The State and the Doctor*, 1910.

231   R Klein, *The New Politics of the NHS,* 6th edition. Radcliffe Publishing, 2010, 280.

232   J McCormick, *The Doctor, Father Figure, or Plumber*, London: Croom Helm, 1979.

233   H Stoate, *The Guardian*, 23 September 2015.

234   B Webb and S Webb, *The State and the Doctor.*

INDEX

A

accidents, 118, 157,158
accoucheur, 60, 71,76
alcohol, 61, 163
Ancient Order of Foresters, 83
annual ball, 160
annual dinner, 101, 210
annual report, 4, 18, 26, 33, 40, 42, 44,
    47, 61, 77, 144, 208
Apothecaries' Act 1815, 212
apothecary, 10, 16, 18, 21, 60, 94 97,
    100, 109, 110, 113, 117, 142,
    160, 170, 184, 228
apprentice, 97, 107, 117, 140, 144, 155
Armstrong, George, 94
Ashmeade, Thomas, 21
asylum, 61, 143, 165

B

bankruptcy, 59
Baretti, TG, 54, 61,73
Bartley, Robert, 77
Beddoe, John, 59, 73, 80
Beddoes, Thomas, 2, 4, 50
beds, 116, 118, 157, 200
Bernard, James F, 77
Blackall, Henry, 162
Boxes, charity, 61
Bright, Richard, 114
Bristol Medical School, 60
Broom, John, 79
British Medical Association, 84,
    119, 202

British Medical Journal, 152,

C

candles, 102, 113, 151
Care Quality Commission, 223
Carter, Thomas M, 62
Carter, William Grover, 73
Chandler, John Moss, 76
charity, 21, 24, 48, 52, 61, 108, 116,
    149, 155
Charity Organisation Society, 192
children, 68, 70, 76, 78, 82, 94, 174,
Challacombe, Peter, 76
Chisholm, Colin, 49, 50, 214
chloroform, 67
cholera, 13, 55, 116, 162
Clark, John, 171
Clifton College, 59
clinical commissioning group, 225
coal, 61, 64, 102. 151
cod liver oil, 118, 147, 193
collector, 101, 114, 117, 144, 199
Colthurst, John, 58, 59
committee, 11, 12, 18, 36-39. 48, 50,
    63, 64, 75, 77, 80, 101, 109, 115,
    117, 144, 148, 155, 163, 194, 201
complaint, 15, 117, 152
convalescent home, 61, 89
Cookson, RG, 64
costs, 21, 67, 97, 100, 118, 142, 177
court cases, 58, 59
consumption, 99, 172, 174

D

typhoid, 1, 115